Change Your Shoes, Change Your Life

Strut Your Way to a Fabulous New You!

Susan Reynolds

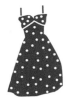

Polka Dot Press
Avon, Massachusetts

Published by Polka Dot Press,
an imprint of Adams Media, an F+W Publications Company
57 Littlefield Street, Avon, MA 02322. U.S.A.
www.adamsmedia.com

ISBN: 1-59337-439-9

Printed in the United States of America.

J   I   H   G   F   E   D   C   B   A

Library of Congress Cataloging-in-Publication Data
Reynolds, Susan (Linda Susan)
Change your shoes, change your life / Susan Reynolds.
p.   cm.
Includes bibliographical references.
ISBN 1-59337-439-9
1. Women—Psychology. 2. Women's shoes—Psychological aspects.
3. Life change events—Psychological aspects. 4. Identity (Psychology).
5. Fashion—Psychological aspects. I. Title.
HQ1206.R456 2005
391.4'13'082—dc22
2005011191

Illustrations by Carlos Marrero.

This book is available at quantity discounts for bulk purchases.
For information, please call 1-800-872-5627.

dedication

I dedicate this book to the memory of my parents:

My mother, Grace Sue Pennington,
whose *southern lady* shoes were difficult to fill.

My father, Roy Joseph Reynolds, who induced me to
fall in love with, and forever don, *vagabond shoes*.

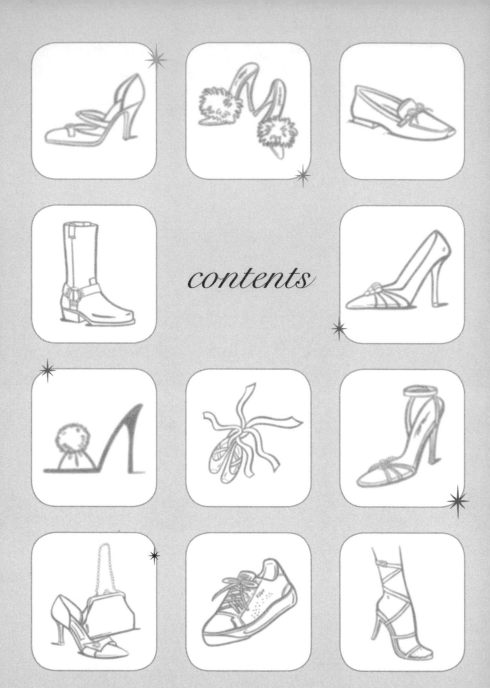

contents

acknowledgments

I would like to thank crucial players in helping this book come to fruition.

In the publishing world: Adams Media for embracing this project; Paula Munier, a visionary, highly talented editor, with a passion for shoes, who assisted greatly in transitioning a simple idea into a complex one; Kirsten Amann, assistant editor and project manager, who coordinated, coaxed, and coached the book through production with great enthusiasm; Carlos Marrero, illustrator, who brought the text to life with imagery; and my agent, June Clark, for her efficient representation and encouragement.

In my personal world: Margie Myers and Kenny Harris, who not only allowed me to use their spare Manhattan apartment to write for eight months when I returned from Paris, but who also supported and encouraged me in making a major life transition; Cristiano Pizzocheri, my young Italian roommate during that time, for always making me laugh when I wanted to cry; Terra Mizwa for truly inspirational guidance; my dear friend, Paula Munier, for her endless years of encouragement and camaraderie; Gale Giorgio for her generous heart; Wanda Whalen for her insightful wisdom; Arlene Corsello for never doubting me, or my resolve; Toni Apgar Thayer for crediting my inventiveness in telling me I was the only one who could make an interesting book out of our shared years at *Footwear News*; Brian Ballerini and his lovely wife, Kirsten Leitner, for welcoming me back to California and lovingly nudging me toward my fate; Sheila Ryan for literally giving me a car to visit libraries and bookstores when I returned to California; my brother, Roy Reynolds, for helping me move on with my life; my champions, Chris and Michele Kaczmarek, for providing backbone when it was sorely needed; my son, Brett, for simply being my son; my daughter, Brooke, for always believing in me and bravely following in my creative footsteps; and all of my contributors. And last, in memoriam, Vivian Infantino, my Fairy Godmother in shoes. Vivian served, most excellently, as the fashion editor for *Footwear News* for more than forty years, during which time she gladly took me—and many others—under her wing. She taught me how to be a fashion editor, how to win promotions at Fairchild Publications, how to leave even when it broke her heart, and how to take great delight in footwear escapades. I will forever remember her, and another former colleague, Mark Perryman, for coloring my early days in publishing.

1

a love affair with shoes

To be carried by shoes, winged by them . . . to wear dreams on one's feet is to begin to give reality to one's dream.

Roger Vivier, French shoe designer

I n France, where so much of fashion originates, the word *chaussures* can mean either shoes or pastry. However, legendary shoe designer Roger Vivier felt so passionately about shoes and how he wanted women to feel when they wore them that he referred to them as *souliers,* or dreams.

While millions of women love shoes and fully recognize their worth in terms of fashion, style, image, and pure pleasure, it's my theory that the great majority of women fall into a psychological chasm when it comes to their shoes, adopting a certain lack of attitude or style that defines them more than they realize. These unfortunate women have failed to realize that changing your shoes can change your life. It all has to do with *strutting your stuff.*

Women who strut their stuff know that the thrill of buying new shoes goes deeper than the adrenaline rush any normal woman experiences when she buys a fantastic new item, be it clothing, a handbag, or shoes. It has more to do with realizing that buying a great pair of shoes revitalizes who you think you are, who you project to others, how you feel about yourself, and even how much fun you're having.

Women who strut their stuff choose their shoes before they pick their outfit. They make shoes the base of their operations, and they buy shoes that make a real statement, whether it's a fashion statement, an image statement, or a sexual declaration.

Women who strut their stuff use fashion statements to say to themselves and to the world that they are women who value their appearance, appreciate quality, change with the times, and possess a certain *je ne sais quoi.* Have you ever slipped on a pair of elegant Chanel slingbacks? Doing so will virtually alter your genetics; you'll feel a tingle go through your feminine bones, and if you walk across the room wearing those shoes, you'll experience a taste of refinement. You can make such refinement your own—without breaking the bank. Thank the Shoe Goddess for inexpensive knockoffs and s*hoe attitude.*

it's a shoe thing

Is a foot just a foot . . . a shoe just a shoe?

So what is the thing with shoes? Sure, they're gorgeous in and of themselves, but shoes are not simple frivolity. In ancient China, for example, footprints stamped onto garments symbolized the wearer's need to be wise when it came to life decisions. In fact, the Chinese ideogram for "foot" is the same as the one for "virtue," indicating the Chinese penchant for linking feet to the higher spirit. Not only do our feet provide balance, stability, and mobility, they also symbolize spiritual flight! If you still don't believe me, consider this: in some ancient cultures, when families buried beloveds, the beloveds were wearing a pair of elaborately decorated slippers, or the slippers were placed within reach. Our best guess: these people believed that fancy traveling shoes facilitated their ascent to

designer dish

Roger Vivier

MASTER SHOE DESIGNER, MANOLO'S PREDECESSOR

Roger Vivier, who studied art in Paris, was the world's premier shoe designer for thirty-five years, including ten years as designer for Christian Dior (1953–1963). Vivier won acclaim for his ornate shoe masterpieces, using glass beads and pearls to almost literally transform shoes into jewelry. His shoes were dress, coat, hairstyle, and jewelry combined; his admirers deemed Vivier shoes "the Fabergé of footwear." For Queen Elizabeth's coronation ceremony in 1950, Vivier designed modified platform shoes in gold kid leather studded with glittering garnets to signify the queen's marriage to her country. Quintessentially French, he created alchemy in style, and many equated owning a pair of Vivier shoes to owning a couturier suit. Classic Vivier shoes are on display at the Costume Institute in the Metropolitan Museum of Art in New York City, the Victoria and Albert Museum in London, and the Musée de la Mode et du Costume at the Louvre in Paris.

heaven. We may not be as focused on the afterlife, but we still love our shoes.

According to Meera Lester, author and shoe enthusiast, shoes frequently play a role in her dreams. "I keep a dream journal and whenever shoes appear, they seem to carry a potent message. Often they symbolize the need to execute a major transformation. They also appear when I'm not feeling particularly grounded or soulful (*soleful*). Sometimes they instruct me to walk away from a bad situation, and sometimes they encourage me to walk straight into a difficult situation and deal with it head-on. I've also had dreams in which shoes were prominent that indicated a need for me to kick out worn-out beliefs or kick up my heels. Dreams in which I am wearing high heels invariably include a drop-dead gorgeous man."

 platitudes relating to shoes and feet

Well-heeled

Down at the heels

Cool your heels

Two left feet

Equal footing

Footing the bill

Put your foot down

Get your foot in the door

Put your best foot forward

You bet your boots

You put your foot in your mouth

Keeps you on your toes

Thinking on your feet

Head over heels

Two steps ahead

Knock your socks off

Kick up your heels

Landing on your feet

Giving someone the boot

You have to walk a mile in his/her shoes

He isn't fit to lick my boots

He can put his boots under my bed anytime

Marie-Louise von Franz, a prominent modern-day psychologist who wrote a fascinating book on fairy-tale interpretation, considered shoes a potent symbol of power, the choice of which directly reflects how we view our current circumstances and our power to alter them for the better. Shoes demonstrate how solidly we plant our feet on the ground of our own beliefs; in turn, how solidly we feel supported gives us the measure of our power. She noted that popular expressions such as "being under someone's heel" or "stepping into your father's shoes" reflect and underscore our primal attachment to shoes.

Other modern-day idioms bear this out: we often counsel our friends that "you need to be on solid ground, standing on your own two feet" before you embark on adventures, including growth-oriented, spiritual pursuits. Once we have embarked, at least in our imagination, it's our feet that take us places. Imagine the Greek god Hermes in his winged shoes, transporting souls to heaven; now imagine an exquisite pair of Christian Louboutin feathered pumps or vintage Roger Vivier shoes trimmed with hummingbird feathers.

Another prominent psychologist, Bruno Bettelheim, believed that myths and fairy tales derived from initiation rites, or other rites of passage, such as the metaphoric death of an old, inadequate self and the adoption of a symbol to represent the birth of a newly reorganized self. In other words, just like Cinderella, when shoes become a metaphor for transformation and you're donning a new pair of shoes, you're giving birth to a whole new you!

So you see, girls, a shoe is not just a shoe. We shod our feet in magnificent shoes because the shoes themselves are the base we stand on, literally and figuratively. Sure, shoes provide stability, comfort, and protection, but they also provide a means for us to tell the world who we are. Even more important, shoes provide divine inspiration to become more than you are or even dream you can be. So the next time someone asks about your teensy shoe obsession, you can legitimately explain that deeply ingrained mythological and psychological needs drive women to develop lifelong love affairs with shoes. Indeed, to view shoes as strictly a utilitarian necessity indicates a cry for help!

shoe-b-shoe-b do

What do your shoes say about you?

Our shoes often are the source of our greatest personal stories. Marjorie Myers, a wholesale shoe representative from New York City, fondly remembers a pair of shoes she bought in 1969. "I had just graduated from college, and like so many of my contemporaries, my boyfriend and I embarked on a summer tour of 'Europe on $5.00 a day.' Because we couldn't find anything substantial enough to hold up to our journey; because we had slaved and saved for a year to accumulate enough money for the trip; and because the dollar was incredibly strong against European currencies at the time, we finally decided to save money by waiting to buy shoes at our first stop in London. Once there, we were delighted to find terrific, sporty, gum-soled leather shoes for me and short, leather chukka boots for him.

"Standing on the roadside, dressed in our *de rigueur* bell-bottom jeans, 5&10-cent-store work shirts, army-surplus jackets, and long-long hair, we looked *trés* international—just like all the Australian, British, Danish, French, and Italian twenty-year-olds trooping around the continent. In fact, to our surprise, not one motorist pegged us as Americans. 'It's your shoes,' they would explain. 'Americans always wear shoes that look like cardboard.' Luckily, in those days, Americans were still the heroes who had saved their countries from disaster in WWII, so they often provided a ride *and* a free place to land for a few days! We not only fell in love with our English shoes, we considered them our *lucky, traveling shoes."*

If you still don't realize how strongly shoes can affect your life, allow me to offer two examples, culled from my own experience, of when shoes have played the starring role.

Two of the most dramatic shoes of my lifetime were my wedding shoes and a pair of high-heeled designer sandals I bought to wear on a pivotal New Year's Eve. On both occasions, I strove for elegance, height, and a sexual purr (as opposed to a sexual come-hither). Because I was a fashion reporter in the shoe business at the time of my marriage, I happened to interview Pasquale Di Fabrizio, a famous shoemaker to the stars, who kindly offered

 fit for a queen

In eighteenth-century Europe, shoes reflected cultural status. Queens wore paper-thin slippers and servants wore wooden *sabots* (clogs). In France, the Empress Josephine once returned a torn pair of her paper-thin slippers to her cobbler, who said "...but Madame, you walked on them."

the ultimate shoe makeover heroine

Dating back to ninth-century China, the Cinderella story appears in more than 700 versions across a myriad of cultures. In the 1800s, a Frenchman named Perrault homogenized the German version, *Aschenputtel*, which Disney then further truncated, eliminating crucial aspects of the fairy tale having to do with Cinderella's transformation. In the Perrault/Disney versions, they portray Cinderella as a wimp! She willingly lives by the hearth, she isn't required to successfully perform impossible sorting tasks, she doesn't symbolically reconnect with her mother's spirit, she isn't aggressive in expressing her desire to go to the ball, she doesn't make a conscious decision to change her fate, and her Fairy Godmother magically grants her wishes anyway. Other versions are much tougher on poor Cinderella, making her rewards seem much more sweet!

to design and handcraft my wedding sandals. He made me an exquisite pair of high-heeled, spaghetti-strapped sandals—simple, elegant, sexy, and marvelously utilitarian. The 3-inch, chunky heels allowed my clinging, sexy, matte-jersey wedding gown to flow over my 5'4" frame and enabled me to literally dance for hours. Di Fabrizio, who had crafted shoes for Sylvester Stallone just before Stallone wrote *Rocky*, told me those shoes would bring me luck, and I believed him; they're still a part of my (very edited) shoe wardrobe.

I bought the second pair of sandals eight years later. By this time, I had given birth to two children, gained 30 pounds, adopted a suburban lifestyle, and was coping with a castigating husband, low self-esteem, and a deepening depression. Along the way, I had somehow discarded Susan—independent, self-possessed, confident, styling, sexy Susan. I had forgotten the importance of gathering myself together and projecting that image to the world. I had, in fact, forgotten the importance of shoes. Luckily, I wandered into a local Nordstrom's where I spied a pair of clear Lucite sandals swathed by a glittering band of rhinestones, teetering on a high, thin, black satin heel. The sandals weren't a *designer*-designer label, but an American shoemaker known for creating wearable art designed and manufactured them. As soon as I slipped those sandals on my feet, I felt transformed. I still remember prancing across the floor, looking in the mirror, and thinking "now, *this* is Susan." I bought myself a gorgeous dress, spent $45 to have my makeup done, added a sassy new haircut, and not only wowed my hypercritical husband, but, far more important, wowed myself that New Year's Eve.

I immortalized those shoes by taking a sexy photograph of them and pasting it into my journal. Those shoes represented a realization that I choose how I feel about myself. Every time I look at that photograph, I feel a positive, strong, sexy, feminine, goddess-like persona coursing through my veins. Buying those shoes and wearing those shoes changed my life. I reclaimed my life and declared myself a woman who knows her own self-worth, whose image of herself comes from the inside out, who embraces her own sexuality, and who isn't afraid to show the world who she is! Like a warrior donning armor, I donned those sandals and felt strong, empowered, sexy, and feminine. I became Joan of Arc in high heels.

cinderella shoes

In fairy tales, shoes are often the vehicle of escape from humdrum lives . . . Clothing (and shoes) may represent either the persona (our outer attitude) or the inner attitude, and the changing of clothes in the mysteries stood for transformation into an enlightened understanding.

Marie-Louise von Franz, prominent psychologist and
author of Interpretation of Fairy Tales

From the time she met her Fairy Godmother to the time she dropped that infamous slipper on the castle steps, Cinderella earned her stripes as poster girl for *shoe attitude*. She maximized the opportunity to *strut her stuff* and wowed a jaded prince in the process. Cinderella's Fairy Godmother understood the allure of shoes and knew that a pair of seductive pumps could play a pivotal role in Cinderella's enchanted evening. She didn't let that girl put one foot into the pumpkin until a fabulous pair of pumps graced her feet. Cinderella's head-to-toe makeover was complete, but it was the discovery of that single, mysterious feminine slipper that spurred the princely quest to find the only woman who could fill those shoes.

In the Grimm Brothers' version, Cinderella began her life privileged. After her father remarried, her stepmother and stepsisters forced her into servitude, gave her a gray dress and wooden shoes to wear, and made her sleep by the hearth. When her father went on a trip and asked what the daughters wanted, the stepsisters wanted diamonds, pearls, and beautiful dresses; Cinderella wanted the first tree branch that brushed against his cheek. She planted the tree branch at her mother's grave and spent so much time tending it and crying that her tears helped turn it into a beautiful tree (representing her internalized "good mother"). A white bird alighted on the branches and rewarded Cinderella by granting her wishes.

When it came time for the ball, Cinderella begged her stepmother for permission to go. The stepmother threw lentils into the hearth and gave her the impossible task of not only finding them all, but sorting them into good and bad lentils. Because she had the white bird on her side, Cinderella asked for all the turtledoves of heaven to help, and they did. When she completed the task, the cruel stepmother made the task even harder, and when Cinderella completed it within the allotted time, her stepmother again denied her the chance to go to the ball. "You have nothing to wear; you don't know how to dance; we would be ashamed of you."

the significance of cinderella's shoes

The beautiful slippers represented Cinderella's ultimate femininity. For the prince, the dainty slipper denoted that which was most desirable in a woman and aroused love for definite, if deeply unconscious reasons. The slipper also represented the solution to the problem of finding his rightful bride. As soon as the prince cherished the slipper, he also cherished Cinderella, so much so that he accepted her femininity, even when he first saw her in her degraded state. When Cinderella purposefully removed the wooden shoe, which belonged to her days at the hearth, and slipped her foot into the proffered golden slipper, the appearance she borrowed for the balls became her true self. The fitting of the shoe symbolized their betrothal.

But the Grimm Brothers' Cinderella did not surrender. After her stepmother and stepsisters left for the ball, she rushed to her mother's grave and cried "Shake your branches little tree. Throw gold and silver down on me." The white bird tossed down a gold and silver dress, and slippers embroidered with silk and silver. (In one of the original versions, Cinderella wore fur slippers; Perrault changed them to glass slippers; the Grimm Brothers described three pairs of increasingly beautiful slippers, with the last, fateful pair being significantly and symbolically golden.) Cinderella arrived at the ball looking so beautiful, they thought she was the daughter of a foreign king; the prince fell instantly in love and thereafter called her "his partner."

At the end of the night, Cinderella chose to hide her true identity. She returned the next night wearing another pair of gorgeous slippers, and the next night wearing golden slippers! On the third night, hoping to forestall her escape, the Prince brushed pitch on the castle steps. When Cinderella left the ball, her golden slipper stuck to the pitch, giving the Prince an opportunity to seek his true bride.

In the traditional version, the stepsisters sliced off parts of their feet to make them fit into the slipper, and it wasn't until the prince and Cinderella's sisters passed the tree and heard the bird announcing "There's blood in the shoe. The foot's too long; the foot's too wide. That's not the proper bride . . ." that the prince realized he had the wrong bride. When he returned the second time, the stepmother told him no one remained except "the kitchen drudge. She couldn't possibly be the bride." The prince sent for her anyway. When Cinderella sat down on a footstool, took her foot out of the heavy wooden shoe her stepmother had forced her to wear, and put it into the golden slipper, it fit perfectly.

shoe do

Because our goal is to change your life through this journey together, we'll offer a *shoe do* and a *shoe date* for each chapter, designed to help you examine and expand your *shoe attitude*. You may want to record your observations in a journal. Your first assignment: Now that we've discussed the importance of *strutting your stuff*, grab a pen and write down the last time you *strutted your stuff* and then describe in detail the clothes you were wearing, focusing, of course, on the shoes. What is it about those shoes that contributed to your empowerment? If you cannot recall the last time you *strutted your stuff*, then we definitely have work to do! Simply record this oversight in your journal so that we'll see how far you've come by the end of our journey. Our motto throughout: no judging, just recording.

When the reunited couple passed the hazel tree, two doves called out "Roocoo, roocoo. No blood in the shoe. Her foot is neither long nor wide. This one is the proper bride." On the day of the wedding, the birds pecked out the stepsisters' eyes (proper retribution that is completely absent in the Perrault/Disney versions).

Why is all this important? Cinderella immortalized the ultimate shoe makeover, but, in the grittier Grimm Brothers' version, she did not achieve this without taking full responsibility for her transformation. This Cinderella had to be wily; she had to transcend her degraded state through a series of tests, including:

* Recognizing her self-worth despite her present conditions
* Discovering aspects of her own personality that would elevate her

* Sorting out good from bad
* Protecting her identity until she was ready to reveal it to the world
* Avoiding surrendering too quickly to her desires
* Knowing that the prince needed to see her in her degraded state and still love her before she could successfully become his bride

Most important, the original Cinderella had to recognize and seize the opportunity to remove her foot from the wooden shoe and place it into the golden slipper. Her reward: the life of grandeur she deserved, and marriage to a prince.

The moral of the story: we transform ourselves from the inside; temporary stages of degradation are not indicative of your true self; entering the lowest depths of existence is but a necessary step toward realization of your highest potential; difficult tasks must be performed

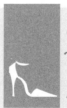

designer dish
Beth Levine

AMERICAN SASS

American footwear designer Beth Levine, created the sexy, stretchy, shiny patent boots that became wildly popular in the 1960s. Levine often designed outside of the box, even using unconventional materials like Astro Turf and frogskin. She won worldwide fame for creating the white go-go boots Nancy Sinatra wore when she performed *These Boots Are Made for Walking* on television.

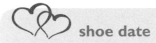 **shoe date**

The idea of a *shoe date* is to find a friend or two to accompany you on your journey of shoe discovery. Think of these friends as your Fairy Godmother(s) of shoes, who will help you define and refine your real shoe destiny. Go ahead, pick up the telephone and invite someone to come along. Arrange to meet for tea to give you an opportunity to present the concept of *shoe attitude* and *strutting your stuff*. Sharing stories will inspire you to delve deeper and result in a substantial step forward. Cheers!

before you are worthy of a happy ending; what exists in reality is less important than what goes on in our mind (when we internalize the good mother); and, if you are true to your inner self, you triumph.

The reason more than 700 versions of Cinderella emerged throughout the world—and survived 1,100 years—is that we are all Cinderella. In other words, we are all born perfect and beautiful, but we all must be prepared to undergo a Cinderella existence, not just in terms of hardships, but in terms of the difficult tasks we each have to master—on our own initiative—to acquire unique personal achievement, individuation, and identity. A huge part of our transformation comes in how we think about ourselves, how we present ourselves to the world, and how we must remove the wooden shoes that weigh us down so that we can slide our feet into our personal, unique, golden slippers to achieve our true identity. By revamping our old images, sorting out the good from the bad, changing the way we think about ourselves, and thereby resolving any underlying, self-sabotaging self-esteem issues, we change our whole lives and reclaim our real destinies.

are you ready, girls?

How many times have you used the expression "you'd have to walk a mile in her shoes"? Walking in someone's shoes means more than knowing what they are going through at the moment; it also means understanding all aspects of their lives—who they think they are, how they feel about themselves, how others view them, how they view the world and their place in it, what they are willing to do or not do, how easy or how hard they've made it for themselves, or even if they're having any fun. Whose shoes have you been walking in? Your grandmother's? Your mother's? Your best friend's? The same shoes you chose when you were seventeen? The shoes you put on when your feet swelled during pregnancy? The shoes you chose for your corporate uniform? The only shoes that don't pinch? Shoes you don't have to think about? Shoes that don't say anything about you? Hooker shoes, athletic shoes, Grace Kelly shoes? *InStyle* pick-of-the-month shoes? Lazy shoes?

In the late 1960s, on the cusp of a feminist resurgence, Nancy Sinatra recorded *These Boots Are Made for Walking*. The lyrics resonated so deeply with women's rising independence that the song became a number one hit. In fact, the lyrics became a femi-nine battle cry, so deeply embedded in our modern mythology that each succeeding generation of girls embraces the song anew. Sure, Nancy and Nancy's sexy little white go-go boots were hot, but, if you're like me, you never put on any pair of boots without feeling (smugly) that you are suited up and ready to walk over anyone who gets in your way.

Sassy boots aren't the only shoes that inspire you to strut. Remember those little pink plastic shoes with teensy-weensy heels and how we tottered around on them, feeling like a princess? Remember begging to wear your mother's high-heeled pumps and how slipping on her "woman" shoes made you feel like a queen? Remember the swagger you developed when you put on the first pair of grown-up high heels you bought by yourself, for yourself? High heels are powerful weapons: they can raise your psyche to the stars and simultaneously lay a man's psyche at your feet. Stiletto heels and sex have become so intrinsically linked, slipping on a pair for five minutes can seriously alter the future of your evening. That's shoe power!

If you aren't *strutting your stuff* to the max, this book is for you! We're going to pry open your fashion psyche, reassess where you are versus where you want to be, define and refine your image, align your private and public image, ransack and revamp your closet, increase your assets, maximize your individuality, teach you how to shake your booty, and change your attitude about life, fashion, and—most of all—you.

Are you ready for your golden slippers?

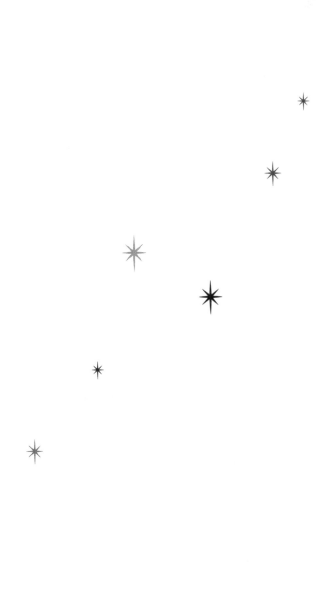

2

the six principles of strutting

I remember walking down the Champs-Elysées. The weather was balmy; it was quite crowded with people, and it was absolutely quiet . . . I can remember exactly what I had on: a little black moiré tailleur from Chanel, a little piece of black lace wrapped around my head, and beautiful, absolutely exquisite black slippers like kid gloves . . . It's curious to visualize yourself like this, isn't it? But I always have to think about what I had on. Just today, I thought about those slippers, and I remembered everything.

Diana Vreeland, fashion icon, longtime fashion editor (Vogue and Harper's Bazaar), and consultant to the Costume Institute at the Metropolitan Museum of New York

before you can properly strut, you have to buy yourself some truly fabulous shoes: shoes that make your heart beat faster, shoes that will magnify your best qualities, shoes that tell the world who you are, shoes that elevate you to the life you so richly deserve. To help you identify your dream shoes, we're going to discuss the Six Principles of Strutting, which are guaranteed to rock your shoe world. It's not math, darlings, it's simply a matter of working the plan. Basically, the six principles are as follows:

six principles of strutting

feet first
Footwear choices do shape your life

your shoe history
Those saddle oxfords and ballet slippers you wore as a little girl may still hinder you and your shoe attitude

i think shoes, therefore i am
Making decisions about your life and incorporating shoes into your action plan

out with the old shoes, in with the new you
Change your shoes and jump-start your career and your love life

shoes make the woman
Revamping your *shoe attitude* to enhance your style, image, and life

strut your stuff
Mastering Shoe Attitude

possible shoe misconceptions

When it comes to shoes, men make their own assumptions.

Types of shoes	What you think it says	What men think it says
Ankle-wraps	I have perfect ankles	I'm into bondage
Athletic	I'm sporty	I don't even think about sex
Boots	I'm a sexy girl	Maybe, but let's see what's under those boots
Clogs	I love anything Danish	I drag my feet and whine
Cowboy boots	I love to two-step	I never wear frilly dresses
Espadrille	I belong on the French Riviera	I expect a life of luxury
Fabric shoes	I'm socially responsible	I can't afford leather
Flip-flops	I'm sooo trendy	I'm cheap as hell
Oxfords	I'm sensible when required	I have my personality locked up
Platforms	I am bold and adventurous	I am petite and overcompensate
Pumps	I'm classic Grace Kelly	I want to be president
Riding boots	I own horses; I play polo	I like horses better than men
Sandals	I have gorgeous feet	I want you to lick my toes
Stilettos	I'm too sexy for my shoes	I'm simply dying to sleep with you

feet first

Footwear choices do shape your life

In general, how we decorate ourselves tells the world who we are. Most notably, it swings from broad to understated. Particularly outrageous clothing, footwear, and accessories tell the world we are flamboyant, spirited, individualistic, unafraid to take huge risks, confident in our personality, and unabashed when it comes to self-promotion. Seriously understated clothing, footwear, and accessories announce to the world that we like to fade into the background, rely on the tried and true, trust others' instincts more than our own, don't have a clue how to express our personality through our wardrobes, and prefer to take the safe route in life.

The great majority of us, however, fall in the middle: Our wardrobe reflects an inkling of our predominant personality muddled by an amalgam of moods. Perhaps your predominant personality is conservative, which means you filled your closet with classic black low-heeled pumps, plain oxfords, expensive leather moccasins, non-ornamented sandals, and white or black athletic shoes. Maybe there's a pair of sexy, stiletto, strappy sandals you wore on your first wedding anniversary (five years ago); maybe there's a pair of rhinestone-studded tennis shoes you bought to attend a David Bowie concert in the '80s; or maybe there's a pair of flowered ballet flats you bought after downing three piña coladas poolside in Mexico.

Or perhaps you've seen yourself as a rocker, and continually select clothes, shoes, and accessories that shocked your mother when you were seventeen. Your closet would probably contain 4-inch-high, funky platforms; thigh-high patent boots with motorcycle zippers; heavily sequined platform sandals; 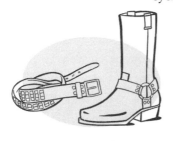 and fluorescent, platform athletic shoes. If you had to attend a funeral, you'd be hard-pressed to find a pair of simple black pumps to wear. There's absolutely nothing wrong with wanting to be a rocker chick, but if you're approaching forty and your job doesn't have something to do with the creative arts, you may be dressing inappropriately and suffering from identity freeze.

Identity freeze occurs when you lock onto a persona—the personality you present to the public—and run with it, even when, in all likelihood, you chose it long before you even knew who you were, and held on to it long after you had outgrown it. While being locked in a rocker chick identity might be painfully obvious, you also can limit yourself by locking into social conservative, miss congeniality, femme fatale, soccer mom, or corporate diva. You get the idea: it's time for an overhaul, but first we have to know from whence we came.

your shoe history

Those saddle oxfords and ballet slippers you wore as a little girl may still hinder you and your shoe attitude

Unless you've gone through some sort of radical transformation, you probably can trace your *shoe attitudes* back to your childhood. If you're like the majority, you're probably emulating a style very close to your mother's. If your mother was demure, you probably dress like Audrey Hepburn and scuttle through life in kitten heels or little black ballet flats. If your mother was an earth-mother who preferred linen baggies and Birkenstocks, you probably don't own a single pair of high-heeled pumps. If your mother insisted on a strict sense of propriety, such as no sandals in the city or no white shoes after Labor Day, chances are you smothered any sense of playfulness and probably don't own a stiletto of any sort. Maybe you learned that shoes were strictly utilitarian.

(Gasp!) Maybe you learned that cheap is perfectly acceptable, or that sensible is the only way to go. Maybe you inherited a truly limited fashion sense, or maybe you didn't inherit any fashion sense at all.

If you don't know exactly what shaped your *shoe attitude*, you'll find the answers by probing deeply into your personal shoe history. You must begin with the first pair of shoes you remember—and why you remember them. For example, I still remember the first pair of shoes that excited me. I was the third daughter and fourth of five children born to a middle-class family within seven years. My parents had neither the time, nor the budget, for fashion; *everything* I owned came down from my sisters. I may have been seven by the time my mother took me to JCPenney to buy my first pair of *real* shoes: creamy white patent Mary Janes, with teardrop cutouts. We lived in South Georgia, and, up to that point, I lived in hand-me-down sandals and bare feet. I do remember how it felt to perch on the leather chair, being the sole focus of a grown-up man, sliding my tiny feet into pair after pair of shoes: delicious. When we agreed upon a pair, I remember staring at my feet admiringly, but also wondering *What am I supposed to do with these?*

"They're your Easter shoes," my mother declared, introducing the concept of special shoes for special occasions and instantly creating a fashion-deprived girly-girl. Although my mother, who exuded southern-lady gentility, traditionally outfitted her daughters in sundresses and clean sandals for Sunday church, she turned Easter into an all-out fashion-fest.

I remember the level of excitement the night before; we spent hours soaking our crinolines in sugar water and standing them in the bathtub to stiffen overnight. I remember our frilly pinafore

dresses and how they puffed out—horizontal to our narrow hips—
when we slipped the crinolines underneath. I remember white
socks with delicately flowered lace, little white gloves with single
fake pearl buttons, a tiny, white patent purse, and a straw sunbon-
net. The creamy white patent Mary Janes were the foundation for
the whole ensemble, and I distinctly remember parading down the
long church aisle in those shoes, feeling very much a princess.

*A beautiful woman is someone who pays a lot of attention
to herself and knows what suits her.*

Vivienne Westwood

That's all very sweet, but the more defining and remarkable part
of my early shoe history is that, prior to buying those Mary Janes,
I had no autonomy. I wore what my sisters wore before me, what
my mother deemed "decent little girl shoes," or what my family
could afford. Because of this, I was a late bloomer when it came to
shoes. My mother often recounted a story about me becoming livid
when a neighborhood bully threw hot tar on my white sandals. As
much as they tried to convince me it meant he liked me, I remained
distraught, evidence that I had a modicum of fashion sense, as well
as a budding *shoe attitude*.

My elder sister took tap and jazz ballet lessons, and I drooled over
her costumes, particularly the silver tap shoes. By the time it became
my turn for tap and ballet, my jaded mother had no interest in indulging my passions. Until I hit puberty, the most memorable shoes I
owned were a pair of brown rubber snow boots topped with a fake

fur collar, purchased when we moved to Pennsylvania and encountered snow for the first time. What I liked best about those boots was that they signaled my new life in what felt like a foreign environment. Wearing those boots linked me to a group of people who talked so fast I couldn't understand them, used odd expressions, dressed entirely different from Georgians, and seemed magnificently exotic.

If it weren't for puberty and my rebellious teenage years, I might still be hampered by southern-lady strictures and live my life seriously footwear deprived. What my girlfriends, or more correctly, what the most popular girls wore set all the style standards, becoming virtually a prerequisite uniform whether or not they made the slightest bit of sense. In my era, cordovan Bass Weejuns for school and little white go-go boots for school dances became the rage. We also wore miniskirts and open-toed sandals in snowstorms, which had the bonus of driving my proper, sane, southern mother crazy. It took eons and threats of utter despair to convince her to buy me my first pair of pink leather, kitten-heel pumps. It was worth the fight: a car full of upper-class boys drove past my junior high school, spotted me *strutting my stuff* in my miniskirt and those groovy pink, kitten-heel pumps, and shouted "nice legs," forever imprinting on my impressionable psyche the value of *shoe attitude.*

As a friend pointed out to me recently, I actually lived a Cinderella life: I went from fashion deprivation to becoming a fashion editor for *Footwear News,* sister publication to *W* and *Women's Wear Daily,* where I spent seven years indulging a newly found shoe obsession and truly learning the value of s*hoe attitude.*

Meera Lester, author and shoe enthusiast, had a similar shoe history. "As the daughter of poor tenant farmers, even though my feet had grown over the summer, unlike luckier girls, I never

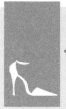

designer dish

Pietro Yantourney

THE ULTIMATE PERFECTIONIST

In the 1920s, Pietro Yantourney, who served as curator of the shoe collection of the Cluny Museum in Paris, became famous for creating custom-made shoes for wealthy women. He began with a plaster cast of the woman's foot and then spent as long as three years perfecting a design, frequently described as "light as cobwebs in extraordinary materials." Even though his customers paid $1,000 a pair (in the 1920s!), he would not permit them to see him or the design until the shoes were completed. His shoes are now on permanent exhibit at the Metropolitan Museum of Art in New York.

got new shoes at the beginning of each school year," she revealed. "Usually a cousin, friend, or another farmer's daughter donated their old pairs. When I won a local spelling bee and needed nice clothes for the countywide spell-off, my mother purchased a deeply discounted pair of shoes that were a size too small. She insisted they just needed to be broken in, but every time I limped to the front of the stage to spell yet another word, the pain in my feet exacerbated the pain in my brain. When I finally misspelled a word, I wasn't devastated; I euphorically collapsed into the nearest chair, gleeful I could sit out the remainder of the competition.

"During my eighteenth summer, I worked as a clerk and window dresser for a department store and finally had the chance to buy my own shoes. I set aside a portion of every paycheck to buy new, correctly fitting shoes *every week*! Confident I was going to be somebody someday, I leafed through trendsetting magazines, searching for footwear that expressed not who I was, but who I wanted to be. I remember discovering fabulous pumps—two-toned, ankle-strapped, sequined sling backs and open-toed, jet black, buttery leather pumps on three-inch heels. Those shoes celebrated my independence, cemented a new image, and catapulted me into adulthood. I've been obsessed with shoes ever since."

Meera's most radical transformation came when she was shopping with her boyfriend's aunt and spied a delicious pair of purple leather pumps with bows. "I salivated over those pumps, but tried to rationalize my way out of buying them, noting that they didn't go with anything I owned. Finally, Steve's aunt said, 'Just get them, darling, you'll find something to wear them with.' It was liberating and all the permission I needed to indulge myself. I bought those pumps, and soon after I married Steve, confident his aunt would support my shoe addiction for life."

I'm nothing to look at, so the only thing I can do is dress better than anyone else.

Wallis Simpson, Duchess of Windsor

Novelist Michelle Cunnah grew up in industrial Sheffield in northern England, where shoes were strictly utilitarian. "Like everyone I knew, I wore the only shoes my family could afford, and I usually owned one, all-purpose, boring pair. Incongruous with my petite frame, I had long, wide feet; nevertheless, I loved shoes and came to believe they held magical appeal. When I was thirteen, chunky, flat, buckled sandals were all the rage. I was convinced those particular sandals would land me a coveted spot with the in-crowd. Begrudgingly, my mother (bless her) bought me a pair. They exaggerated the size of my long, wide feet and were painful to wear, but I wore them relentlessly!

"Unfortunately, this engendered a pattern of stuffing my size 8½ wide feet into narrow, fashion shoes. I adored the Cinderella myth, and soon linked finding the right shoes with finding the right man, and then spent years searching for the right fit on both counts. Like many women in the 1980s, I went through a long line of bad shoes and disastrous men.

"When I finally met Prince Charming, he insisted the size of my feet was fine and encouraged me to choose comfortable shoes that fit over fashionable shoes simply for the sake of fashion. Not long after we married, however, I spied a pair of *very* expensive, femi-nine, low-heeled, highly fashionable, black suede pumps and fell madly in love with them. Although I hesitated, my husband urged me to try them on. In the right size, they not only slipped on easily, they made me feel divinely sexy. My prince bought me those shoes, touching my heart so deeply, twenty years later, I wove this same plot line into a novel, *Confessions of a Serial Dater* (HarperCollins/Avon, August 2005). Like me, my heroine searches frantically for a pair of *Cinderella shoes,* and while I don't want to give away the ending, let's just say it all works out beautifully."

So now that Meera, Michelle, and I have mapped out our his-tories, it's time to delve into *your* shoe history and delineate where your *shoe attitude* and habits of dressing originated. Did you auto-matically dress like your mother? Your favorite aunt? Your grand-mother? Your best friend? Your high-school cheerleaders, the campus rebels, 1980s rock stars, or classic movie stars? Do you have a long history of buying conservative shoes in brown or black and little else? Do you love shoes and see them as the greatest form of personal expression ever created? Or have you been trapped into thinking of shoes as a not-so-important afterthought?

If you don't already possess a *shoe attitude*, you need to develop one in order to jump-start your life through footwear. We begin by living, breathing, and thinking shoes.

i think shoes, therefore i am

Making decisions about your life and incorporating shoes into your action plan

Before you can create the life you want—or create the shoe wardrobe of your dreams—you have to think about your aspirations and map out a strategy. Have you been wishing and hoping for a new life? In fairy tales, the main cause of any event is a wish. When their current circumstances are miserable, fairy-tale heroines wish to magically trade their old life for a new life—one they have imagined to be far better. Although Walt Disney led us to believe that Fairy Godmothers appear to magically grant fairy-tale wishes, the truth is that even fairy-tale heroines, including our poster girl, Cinderella, are required to perform difficult tasks—particularly releasing old identities and forging new ones—before their wishes come true. Still, far too often, we base our wishes on magical, mystical, infantile thinking. A friend of mine, who is also a fabulous therapist, used to crow "I'm waiting for my real mother and father, the Queen and King, to show up and magically transform my life." *As if . . .*

Desires or wants, on the other hand, are real and offer their own fulfillment. When you desire something, you know what you want, which means you are ready to outline and set in motion the steps necessary to get it. You also can choose to deny your own desires and remain unsatisfied, but either way, declaring your wants is entirely different from wishing. "I wish you would stop bothering me" is not nearly as effective as "I *want* you to stop bothering me." Clearly defining, expressing, and fulfilling your wants and desires creates greater potency and energy than wishing and hoping for something to magically change.

A major difference also exists between choice and decision. We make choices every day: what time to get up, what to wear, what to have for lunch, what book to read, and when to go to bed. Most choices involve a goal we can easily fulfill. We choose to arise early so that we can get to work on time; we choose to wear flat, heavily cushioned shoes to the museum so that we don't damage our feet by walking on marble floors for five hours.

I like women to see my shoes as objects of beauty, as gems outside the realm of fashion, within their own universe. Shoes are not an accessory; they're an attribute. You should open a shoebox as if opening a present. Voilà!

Christian Louboutin, shoe designer

Decisions usually involve something that is paramount to our future happiness: we make the decision to fall in love; we make the decision to change careers; we make the decision to move to a new city. Often we cannot predict the outcome, but we make our decisions based on what we know about the world, what we know about ourselves, what we feel deeply within, or what others have counseled us to pursue. Even though our decisions are often life-altering, we may not have a real clue about why we are making them. We decide to follow a certain path because somehow we know that doing otherwise will betray something critical to our very being. Usually, we feel—deep in our bones—that we must take this course of action, no matter the consequences.

So here's the thing, girls: Even, or especially, when it comes to shoes, you need to think about your choices and empower yourself to make footwear choices that help you to catapult your life to new heights.

out with the old shoes; in with the new you

Change your shoes and jump-start your career and your love life

When it comes to revamping your *shoe attitude* and thereby revamping your life, you need to take a series of concrete steps to define, express, and pursue your desires, wants, and dreams. Once you have outlined what it is you want and determined ways in which you can achieve it, you need to make potent choices and decisions.

For example, if you want to move up in your career, it may be time to change your image from a mouse to a pit bull. Often, choosing a shoe wardrobe that sends a message of competency, assertiveness, and confidence will catapult your career from ground zero to the glass ceiling. Shoes are crucial because they are the base upon which you make your stand. Just think about what we know about businessmen: they evaluate other men by the shoes they wear—using qualifiers such as quality, style, cost, and grooming as indicators of the man's social status, business acumen, and forceful personality. No man in worn-out, scuffed, nondescript, terribly out-of-date, black lace-up oxfords gets to the top.

You also can quickly transform a flagging love life through footwear choices. If you've been wearing raggedy old beachcombers around the house, imagine your lover's surprise when you wear the same tattered pair of cigarette jeans but don a pair of sexy red pumps! The poor dears usually sweat, beg, and lie down on command.

Those choices can transform aspects of your life, but making a decision to revamp your entire image can *change* your life. Breaks with the past create a revolution, and a revolution usually spawns art, creativity, and innovation. Are you ready for a personal revolution? If you're not sure, consider this list of concrete reasons to jump-start your image:

* You haven't changed your look in five years.
* You rarely receive compliments on your fashion sense.
* Your boss consistently passes you over for promotions.
* You still haven't attracted the kind of man you want.
* Your sex life is virtually nonexistent.
* Your whole life has recently changed.
* Your closet is not in harmony with your life.
* You aren't expressing who you really are.
* Your closet has too many *someday* clothes or *if only* clothes.

shoe do

You really do have homework to do, darlings. Retrieve your journal from its hiding place and then sit down somewhere comfy. Now, think back to the first pair of shoes that made your little heart trill and march forward, pausing to reflect on each of pair of significant shoes in your life and what they represented to you. Write it all down, darlings. If you find that you've never given real thought to the emotional value of shoes, I want you to imagine a pair of shoes that would make your heart trill and then write a brief, detailed description. Anything goes! Not only will this will help you develop *shoe attitude*, it will shine a light on your emerging persona, thereby putting your feet solidly on the transformation path.

shoes make the woman

Revamping your shoe attitude to enhance your style, image, and life

A great pair of shoes complements silhouette and wardrobe, elevating everything else in an outfit . . . Shoes reveal more about your taste level and eye for detail than any other accessory . . . It's tougher to 'fake it' with cheap shoes than any other item in your wardrobe.

Kendall Farr, author of The Pocket Stylist

La premiere French couturier Coco Chanel once quipped that perfume was "the unseen, unforgettable, ultimate accessory of fashion . . . that heralds your arrival and prolongs your departure." When it comes to style, however, shoes are visible accessories that definitely leave a lasting impression. Shoes reflect your self-image, your priorities, your confidence, your goals and expectations, even your attitudes about sex. Shoes are literally the base you stand on, the most pivotal accessory in your entire wardrobe. They reveal more about your taste level and sense of style than any other item in your wardrobe. They are also gorgeous, titillating, sensuous, electrifying, and offer fabulous opportunities to express your individuality. Consider them precious gems that provide fashion clarity and pizzazz, as well as the image of value, sophistication, elegance, and wealth.

Even if you're not a glam seeker, you still want, as all women do, to radiate beauty, grace, and confidence. You want your clothes

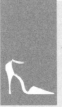

designer dish

Diana Vreeland, high priestess of fashion

FASHION EDITOR OF *HARPER'S BAZAAR,* EDITOR-IN-CHIEF OF *VOGUE,* FASHION CURATOR

The French described their American fashion idol, Diana Vreeland, as *jolie laide* (beautiful ugly). A plain woman who literally transformed herself through fashion, she married a handsome man, and, thanks to her forceful personality, superb taste, and indomitable spirit, dominated fashion journalism for fifty years. She garnered a reputation for fierce fashion discernment. When she took over at *Vogue,* the staff braced for a total magazine makeover. Instead, D.V., as she was called by admirers, stopped wearing her trademark snoods, stopped dyeing her coal-black hair navy blue, cropped it very short instead, and starting wearing cashmere sweaters and skirts in brilliant colors. She also painted her office red, and then she set about reinventing *Vogue.* Her high work ethics, insatiable curiosity, and originality made her a standout in anyone's book. When *Vogue* fired her in 1971, she triumphed as curator for the Costume Institute at the Metropolitan Museum of New York, where her popular exhibits drew more than a million visitors.

to reflect everything positive about you, your inner and outer attributes, your unique gifts, and your resources. Ideally, your shoe wardrobe will reflect your deepest desires and your most cherished images of yourself. If you develop a *shoe attitude* and amass a shoe wardrobe that maximizes these attributes, you'll create an image that becomes your very own public service announcement—*here's who I am, here's how much I value myself, here's how sexy I think I am, here's how successful I believe I am, here's how well I put everything together, here's me being me.*

Diana Vreeland—fashion icon, longtime fashion doyenne, and perhaps our all-time *shoe attitude* heroine—built her entire image on her sense of style. Her husband, Reed, understood her penchant for fashion and patiently indulged her shoe obsession. One famous story originated when they were leaving the Isle of Capri during World War II. Reed boarded a ship bound for America, leaving

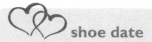 **shoe date**

Invite your Fairy Godmother(s) over for more delicious tea (or cocktails). Take turns imagining that you walked into a room of strangers. Based solely on visual cues—what you're wearing and how you walk into the room—have each person write down the words they think 75 percent of these strangers would employ to describe you. What would they deduce based on your posture, grooming, clothing, accessories, hairstyle, and shoes? If you're not happy with the results, you've been hiding things about yourself, and only one real question remains: Are you ready to show the world the real you? If the answer to that question is a resounding "yes," congratulations—you're ready for a brand-new *shoe attitude.*

Diana behind in war-torn Paris. When friends expressed dismay, he reportedly said, "There's no point in taking Diana away from Chanel and her shoes . . . if she hasn't got her shoes and her clothes, there's no point in bringing her home. That's the way it has always been and that's the way it will always be."

strut your stuff: mastering shoe attitude

What one is is nothing. What one seems to be is everything.

Jean Jacques Rousseau, philosopher

Now that you've decided to change your shoes and change your life, it's important to remember that the whole point is to uplift yourself, to be the best you can be, to walk through the world with your essence on display, your confidence in your pocket, and your fanny swaying. You want to live, breathe, walk, talk, and exude *shoe attitude.* That is, you want to create an image that fits who you are, who you want to be, who you want others to see, and who makes you feel the best about yourself. Once you have that look defined, refined, and collectively on-board, it's time to *strut your stuff*—that is, walk the walk and talk the talk.

We all have gone through many phases in our lives, phases when we sparkled, feeling strong, focused, positive, motivated, energized, magnetic, and sexy—and phases when we hid from the world, feeling depressed, discouraged, exhausted, frustrated, unhappy, and impotent. I don't know how you handle the down times, but when I am in the low-level phase, I tend to gain weight (the perfect way to hide in this thin-obsessed culture), become lethargic, stay home a lot, and put little to no effort into how I look or what I wear. When I decide I have had enough and it's time to turn my life around, I launch a makeover, beginning with a sassy haircut, followed by a wardrobe makeover (brighter colors, bolder fashion statements, a leather jacket, and a killer pair of shoes). Within days of the attitudinal shift and accompanying style makeover, I walk around feeling pumped up, recharged, rejuvenated, refreshed, toughened, sharp, witty, wise, and sexy as hell.

My daughter, Brooke, who has been invaluable at blasting me out of the low-level phases and nudging me in exploratory directions during the high-level phases, used to tell me that I needed to

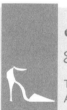

designer dish

Elsa Schiaparelli (1890–1973)

THE "ANTI-CHANEL" FRENCH CLOTHING AND ACCESSORY DESIGNER

Elsa Schiaparelli, a darling of the art world, collaborated with Dali, Picasso, and Man Ray. She fell in love with emerging American sportswear, but added twists, such as buttons in the form of sugar cubes or bugs. Katherine Hepburn, Greta Garbo, and Joan Crawford were among her fans. When shoe designer Roger Vivier sketched fuchsia platform boots in 1937, his employer nixed them as "too radical" for inclusion in his line. Ever the vanguard, Elsa Schiaparelli commissioned Vivier's designs for her next collection, and platforms became all the rage in the 1940s. Schiaparelli loved bold colors and bold designs, often in juxtaposition to her rival, Coco Chanel. Shocking Pink became not only her signature color, but the name of her trademark lipstick and perfume.

dress myself up, go to our local Target, and simply let men look at me. I would always laugh, but Brooke was right. When I felt great about the way I looked—which I created by highlighting all of my assets and buying clothes that strengthened rather than hid them—I could *strut my stuff* anywhere and turn heads.

You can do this no matter your age or who you are; you're never too young or too old to *strut your stuff*. For example, I recently went out with a very attractive, seductively attired, exceedingly thin friend two decades younger than I. When we walked into a local jazz club, heads turned . . . *toward me*. And friends, it had everything to do with what I was wearing—a pair of pin-striped, beautifully cut, low-rise, flare trousers from Paris; a beautifully cut, understated, windowpaned beige (so I could shine) silk blouse, accented with a contrasting, subtly flowered voile shawl; and a pair of navy blue, fabulously fake alligator oxfords (understated yet possessing enough fashion pizzazz to say *she's got a shoe attitude*).

Over the course of the next few weeks, whenever my young friend returned solo, she reported that several men asked, "Who *was* that dynamic woman you were in here with a few weeks ago?" She demanded to know my secret. "Honey," I said, "I wore an outfit that maximized my assets, conveyed who I was and how I was feeling about myself. I walked into that club feeling empowered, attractive, fashionable, and, yes, even at my age, hot—my *Susan light* was shining and when I allow that little light to shine it is consistently, marvelously magnetic."

Girlfriends, it comes down to this: It's all about having *shoe attitude*. In the next chapter, we're going to creak open your closet door to take a close look at your *shoe attitude*, assessing where you've been and determining where you want to go. But before we launch into our master plan to change your life, rush out to your local music store and buy yourself a copy of Patti Labelle singing *New Attitude*. Come home, slap it on your CD player, hit the repeat button, jump up and down, and sing along with me—*I've Got a Shoe Attitude*!

3

everybody out of the shoe closet

Even when we wear nothing, our clothes are talking noisily to everyone who sees us . . . unless we are naked and bald, it is impossible to be silent.

Alison Lurie, author of The Language of Clothes

by now you understand why it's good to review and revamp your shoe habits, so let's get to work. Like Cinderella, you have some sorting to do. We've discussed how easy it is to fall into habitual dressing and how you may be clutching old attitudes about yourself and your style to your chest. Maybe it's been eons since you stepped out of your comfort zone and took a footwear risk; maybe you've *never* explored options or bought a pair of shoes simply to counter every image you've held of yourself.

Well, girls, no regrets and no chastising. Our only purpose in looking backward is to ferret out

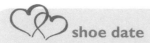

shoe date

Cleaning out your closet is always more fun when your Fairy Godmother comes along. In fact, she'll be the one who offers the most salacious input, so offer the poor darling a small pitcher of vodka martinis and listen to everything she says. In fact, write it down! When you don't have the heart to cull shoes from your life, let her do the honors. You'll thank her later.

old patterns, discard everything that's no longer working, and map out a strategy to expand your wardrobe, your image, your social life, your professional life, your sex life, and your capacity for fun. From now on, we're forging new territory. If you want to *strut your stuff* and change your life, you have to do the work. Are you ready to roll up your silk stockings and talk shoes?

To begin, pull every shoe you own out of your closet. Yes, pull *every shoe* out of the closet—leave no pair unturned—and line them up on the floor. If you like, return them to their original boxes. If the boxes aren't already marked, get yourself a Sharpie and neatly write which shoes go into which box. (We'll cover closet organization in later chapters.)

Now, I want you to group your shoes into broad categories:

Dressy   Shoes for weddings, evenings out on the town, the opera, the theater, the symphony, church, an elegant party, a hot date, afternoon tea with your girlfriends, PTA meetings, or tango lessons

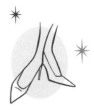

Casual   Includes shoes that are moderately dressy *and* the opposite of dressy; most flats, loafers, sandals, or oxfords

Work   Shoes that complement whatever your particular *work uniform* happens to be

Boots   All boots, be they fashionable, dressy, casual, equestrian, cowboy, line dancing, motorcycle, snow, or rain

Sports/Athletic   Shoes for hiking, sneakers for running errands, running shoes, walking shoes, jogging shoes, workout shoes, ballet slippers, golf, tennis, or bowling shoes

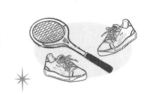

Okay, take a few moments to review the whole stash. Trends may already be painfully evident: you are way overstocked on casual and don't have one single pair of hot date shoes; you don't own a pair of high heels; the only pair of boots you own are seriously out-of-date; your athletic shoes are all deadly boring; your work shoes are all brown or black; or your casual shoes reflect a big, fat fashion zero.

Now, group your categories according to function and price range (over $100, $50–$100, and under $50) so that you can literally see your buying trends in terms of how much you're willing to spend in each category and also in terms of specifics. Consider how many pairs of hot date shoes you own versus how many pairs of afternoon tea shoes you own; how many work shoes you own

and you think you own too many shoes!

Marie Antoinette had a maid whose sole purpose was tending to Madame's 500 pairs of shoes.

Estimates ran as high as 3,000, but according to Imelda Marcos, she actually owned 1,060 pairs of shoes.

In the 1940s, Joan Crawford owned 300 pairs of pumps.

Bombshell Jayne Mansfield owned 200 pairs of pumps.

Soul Diva Patti Labelle admits to owning 4,000 pairs of shoes!

versus how many you need; how many pairs of runaround sneakers you own versus cute sandals to show off your feet. Have you neglected the dressy category altogether? Are you stuck in a rut when it comes to one particular look?

Now, the fun part. It's time to play anthropologist.

what your shoes really say about you

A rich man's wife wears Armani, but his mistress wears Versace.

Teri Agins, author of <u>The End of Fashion</u>

Now that you've separated your shoes into specific, defining categories, you'll be able to gain an accurate picture of your *shoe attitude* by taking an overall look and recording your findings. Recording is an important part; it's so easy to forget what you've learned, and so easy to slide right back into familiar patterns.

To figure out where you've been in relation to where you want to go, sift through your shoes as if they were artifacts. It helps to imagine that the shoes belong to an unknown woman from a foreign culture, and you are a scientist trying to describe the woman who owns them in terms of her habits, her taste, and her image. You don't literally have to turn every shoe over in your hands, but if you want to, particularly to relive emotional attachments—releasing any that are negative and celebrating the positive—please do so. Remember, extra time and effort spent on this sorting task (keep in mind that Cinderella didn't get to the ball without sorting) will pay off down the road. Spend time, look closely—avoid averting your eyes from the unpleasant truth, and celebrate any evidence of an integrated sense of style—but, above all, be specific and brutally descriptive.

Suggested questions include the following.

Are you experiencing déjà shoe?

Do you own a broad spectrum of shoes or do you tend to buy the same shoe over and over? A black leather pump is a black leather pump is a black leather pump. Just as you can endlessly buy black slacks, neglecting opportunities to add real spice to your wardrobe, you can endlessly buy black, mid-heel pumps, creating a classic, if somewhat dull, image.

Where does the money go?

Do you have a few expensive shoes? A plethora of inexpensive shoes? A fair number of moderately priced shoes? No value judgments here! Just use simple observation to determine if your system works . . . or does a plethora of inexpensive shoes (cheap, really) indicate that you lack self-esteem?

Do you have too many or too few shoes?

Okay, you can never have too many, but you can have way, way, way too few. Or you may have too many substandard shoes, in which case trading up may be in order.

Is your shoe wardrobe seriously out of balance?

If yes, which specific categories are overweighted? Under-weighted? If you're single and there's not a single pair of hot shoes in your wardrobe, what do you think that says about your sex life? If you're a lawyer but there's not a single pair of casual shoes in your wardrobe, are you letting your whole life revolve around work? If you're a young mother and you don't own a pair of running shoes, you're going to need a pair when the baby starts to walk!

Are you contemporary or terribly out of date?

Contemporary means that you bought a great pair of shoes in the last three months and the bulk of your shoes within the last two years; terribly out-of-date means you haven't bought a decent pair of shoes in five years—hard to believe, but it happens!

Do you prefer high heels or low heels?

Again, this is not a value judgment, simply an indicator of what works for you. This will be an integral part of developing your *shoe attitude* later.

Do your shoes show a flair for fashion or design?

Designer shoes earn a big plus in this category, but interpretations also count! So do embellishments, unusual colors or stunning color combinations, fabric experimentation, cleverly incorporated patterns, innovative styles, *avant-garde* heels, overall diversity, and so on.

Do you have a distinctive style or project a clear image?

We'll be revisiting this question over and over throughout the book. We are, after all, developing a *shoe attitude* that displays your unique style and projects whatever image you want to project in every circumstance. Usually, it's a shock to find out your shoe wardrobe is far more lackluster than you imagined. Maybe you thought you were quite the femme fatale, but you can't find two pairs of shoes that make your blood rush! Or maybe you're a pop star, and you don't own a single platform. Oops!

Do you regularly update and edit your wardrobe?

If not, no worries—that's exactly what we're working toward.

After your preliminary research is completed, it's time to make critical deductions—critical as in discerning, not judgmental. After scientific scrutiny, what can you tell me about the woman who owns all those shoes spread across the floor?

Do you have a strong self-image?

If yes, your notes should be able to help you pinpoint who you are: You are a professional woman with a variety of interests; you maintain your vitality through vigorous sporting activities; you love to dress up and go out on the town and see yourself as sexually vital; you dance the tango on weekends; you like to spice up your life with color and drama.

Do you hold yourself in high self-esteem or low self-esteem?

You buy only the best and maintain your clothing and shoes so that you'll always look the way you feel: powerful, polished, stylish, and worth every penny.

Do you care about how you look?

You definitely care about how you look: your closet is full of designer shoes; your shoes all reflect a strong sense of style; your shoes coordinate with your clothes beautifully.

Who is the woman behind the shoes?

Do you see yourself as a conservative lady, a fashion plate, a hottie, a nun, a matron, a teenager, a grandma? Does this image fit with who you are? Diversity is a good thing and rigidity is a bad thing in terms of self-image; start making a list of looks you need to buy to expand your vision of yourself.

Do you have a secret side?

Or even a fetish? Nothing wrong with that whatsoever, if you feel inclined to indulge yourself occasionally. If your sex life has been a sleeper, a fetish for silk stockings and Manolo Blahnik stilettos could be a healthy way to shake the blahs (pun intended).

Do you value sex appeal?

If you do, and your closet is sadly lacking sexy shoes, that's a clear rallying cry for some serious shopping ahead. You'll want to think total packaging: sexy dresses, silk stockings, garter belts, and perfume.

Do you go out much?

If you've stopped buying shoes to step out in, you need to get a grip, run to the nearest shoe store, and start plotting a new life. Buy the shoes and the social life will come.

Do you make an impression at work?

If the closet is full of low to medium-height stacked heel pumps, you're not working hard enough to project a power-player image. Score points for conservatively styled pumps in bold, fringe colors and varied textures, like pumpkin suede, electric blue alligator, or red leather.

Does anyone notice you?

If all the shoes in the closet are dull, you need to get out of the closet and gaze into the mirror. Look hard, and start imagining how it would feel if everyone looked at you admiringly.

Does everyone think you're older than you really are?

Yikes! All too often women give up on fashionable shoes way before their time. Sure, we've all got to lower the heel heights as we age, but you can still find fabulous shoes, in fabulous colors, with a great deal of style pizzazz. I know you're coloring your hair; when it comes to finding sexy shoes, work harder!

Do you need to treat yourself to some great shoes?

This is the fun one. Of course you do!

When my friend, Linda, called me over for a shoe consultation, we pulled her shoes out of her closet and went through them one by one. Linda is a gorgeous, sexy, vital woman who had lost her way. While she still radiated those qualities, her shoe wardrobe was sadly lacking and did nothing whatsoever to reflect her true personality. She hadn't bought a new pair of shoes in more than two years and had fewer than fifteen pairs of well-worn, nondescript, functional shoes in her entire wardrobe. Her closet held four pairs of very plain, black leather slip-ons, a pair of clunky brown clogs, a scuffed pair of black, slouchy boots, two medium-heel summer sandals, a pair of thong sandals, a pair of comfort sandals, and a few pairs of white sneakers, all of which she either owned for years or bought at a local discount store. Linda had shoved the two pairs of sexy high-heeled shoes she owned to the back of the closet. Because she no longer worked in an office, she had jettisoned whatever remained of her classic pumps

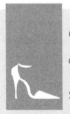

designer dish

Guccio Gucci

SADDLE UP!

As a youth Guccio Gucci worked at the Savoy Hotel in London, where he noticed and admired the luscious leathers and bold ornamentation that defined expensive luggage. When he returned to Florence, he began making leather bags and shoes using horse snaffles. Today, Gucci's classic designs are so *de rigueur* it's one of the few shoe lines that actually have waiting lists for new designs. Most outrageous shoes: crocodile slingbacks.

and had not replaced them with any sharp dress-up shoes. Linda admitted that she had lost interest in dazzling her husband and had increasingly grown complacent about taking care of herself.

This attitude had factored into every aspect of her life. Linda didn't exercise regularly, didn't treat her skin to facials, have her hair cut and styled by a trendy salon, or even buy herself new clothes often. She remained an extremely attractive woman, but she had almost literally gone underground. When she looked at her shoes in light of what they said about her she exclaimed, "I'm so boring!"

The qualities I find sexy in a person include intelligence, humor, and really good shoes.

Sting, rock star

Linda needed to totally rejuvenate her shoe wardrobe, so we began by creating her desirable *shoe attitude*. Linda quickly realized she both needed and wanted to focus much more energy on herself, including pampering herself physically and spiritually. I asked her to delineate specifics: Did she want to schedule regular spa visits? Did she want to work with a personal shopper to build a wardrobe? Did she want to join a gym and work with a personal trainer? Did she want to book regular date nights with her husband? Did she want to plan weekend getaway trips and surprise him with her sexy new image?

As we worked toward a clear image of what Linda wanted her life to reflect about her, I asked her to write a brief description of a woman she admired and how that particular woman's style of dress reflected her personality. In doing so, Linda realized that the

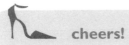
cheers!

In the cocktail culture of the 1970s, art historian and shoe designer Andrea Pfister created a shoe balanced on a martini-glass heel filled to the brim with booze, sporting a bobbing olive.

women she admired maintained an interest in how they looked to the rest of the world. They wore coordinated, dressier outfits, such as silk blouses, trousers, and medium-heeled pumps for trips to the grocery store, donned sexy black dresses and high-heeled, rhinestone sandals for dates, and wore jazzy sneakers for workouts.

We pretty much tossed everything Linda owned and compiled a wish list of clothing and shoes she wanted to start acquiring. Because sprucing up her sex life felt paramount, we began by pulling out whatever dresses or skirts she had in her wardrobe that would inspire her to dress up. Once we selected the keepers, we discussed shoe styles that would perfectly complement the outfits and leafed through fashion magazines to find examples.

In terms of dressing up her daily life, we built our plan around purchasing a few pairs of classic trousers, a few sweater sets, a few silk blouses, and a few skirts. For these, Linda wanted stylish, yet comfortable shoes. She settled on a pair of black patent, reptile print loafers on a small, stacked heel and a pair of 1-inch-heeled sandals with a broad cross-band in supple brown leather. For casual wear, she wanted a pair of trendy striped trainers to put a spring in her steps, and a pair of brown soft-leather, front-zip, ankle boots on a thick rubber sole.

And thus began Linda's shoe makeover. Once she appropriately adjusted her *shoe attitude* and defined her specific needs, the task of transforming her image was well under way. Linda made a clear and exciting choice to step back into the limelight, to take on the starring role in her own life. Now that she knew who she wanted to be, all she had to do was dress the part.

what you want your shoes to say about you

When I'm in Armani, I don't feel that I'm somebody else. It's important that his clothes makes me look better but enhance who I am. The clothes focus on you.

Glenn Close

If this process is working, you now have a much better idea of the image you've been projecting and whether or not it's the image you want to project. Without berating or criticizing yourself (really girls, there is absolutely no point to self-flagellation), own it, as they say, and move on. Provided you've done your homework, your very own Fairy Godmother of shoes will whisk her wand over your tousled head, grant you a pardon, prescribe five scouting trips to Macy's, Saks, Bergdorf's, or Nordstrom's, and give you a second chance.

But not before you read every word you recorded and truly learn your lessons!

Okay, confession is over. It's time to map out a strategy for the new you! You've probed your past, questioned your motivations (or lack thereof), and documented your fashion *faux pas* history. Let's take all this information and flip it!

What is the primary image you want to project in each area of your life? If you want to project a fashion image and your current wardrobe is seriously lacking, you need to make a shopping list. *Hint*: Whenever you're leafing through a magazine, rip out pictures of shoes that intrigue you or that you need in your closet. Create a dream or *wish book* of desired items—broken down into categories—and paste the pictures in their respective categories. (More on this in Chapter 9: The Master Plan.)

What's your dating image? If you haven't been dating often or if your last Valentine's Day present was a toaster, you may need to add some high heels, sexy slingbacks, or mules. If you've been operating as a wallflower and you want to make a man's blood boil, red or fuchsia stiletto sandals could spin you into a new strato-

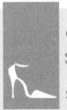

designer dish

Salvatore Ferragamo

SHOEMAKER TO THE STARS

At age nine, Salvatore Ferragamo designed and handcrafted his first pair of shoes. His sister's first communion was approaching, and he didn't want her to have to wear wooden *sabots*, considered peasant shoes at the time. By age sixteen, he recognized that he had a talent for shoe design and ambitiously immigrated to Hollywood, where he became shoemaker to the stars. He designed cowboy boots for Gene Autry, dance pumps for Mary Pickford, and boudoir sandals for Gloria Swanson. Later, he innovated steel arch supports to distribute women's weight, thereby allowing them to wear high heels more comfortably.

shoe do

Now that you've wallowed in the bitter truth, or celebrated your total fabulousness, select your "playing it safe" shoes and your "taking a chance" shoes. Do a little soul searching in your journal, specifically asking yourself what both kinds of shoes say about your personality. End by making a list of qualities you want to generate, and jot down any ideas for shoes that will pave the way.

sphere. If you've been dressing like a nun, over-the-knee suede boots paired with a miniskirt could change your life. If you've been a flat-heeled, slip-on girl, feminizing your footwear could lead to interesting developments. The more you feel like a sexy woman, the greater the chances he'll treat you like a sexy woman. Remember, girls: you were born to *strut your stuff!*

Now take a look at your professional image. If your coworker stole the last promotion right out from under your classic pumps, it may be time to strengthen your power image. I'm not suggesting you go wild, but red is a power color. Why not wear red shoes? If you've been skating by on inexpensive shoes with zero fashion, get a grip. Those who dress rich, get rich.

In the casual and athletic categories, I'll wager that, if you're like 80 percent of the female population, a lack of imagination has stunted your repertoire. In what has traditionally been a deadly boring category, there is no longer any excuse for slacking given the vast array of styles available today. Track suit or no track suit, expensive shoes make a definitive statement; fashion shoes make a personality statement; contemporary shoes make a hip factor statement.

We're going to home in on these areas and dig much deeper into specifics later, but please take another overview and carefully note where your strengths and weaknesses lie. What areas in your wardrobe need serious expansion? What areas are overstocked? What specific items do you need to change your image, your attitude, your sass factor, your life?

the truth be soled

At this stage, we've constructed a wide-angle snapshot of who you've been up to now. Farther down the road, we'll focus on wardrobe preening and wardrobe building. Nevertheless, we're ready to make quick, painless cuts—no whining, no hesitating, and absolutely no excuses. We're cleaning up your life, girlfriend. Be ruthless; be the Athena of closet reorganization. Take a deep breath, head over to the dressy category, and work your way through each subcategory, eliminating shoes as follows.

Old Shoes

If shoes are seriously out-of-date, pitch them. That old cliche about styles always coming back is simply not true. Sure, Louis heels, needle toes, and platforms come back (like a bad penny), but *never* in the same way and rarely in the same materials. If you covet and would genuinely wear funky, vintage shoes, and you have a few spectacular pairs in quality materials that also are in great shape, then by all means keep them. But if you're holding on to a category because you think they'll look trendy some time in the future, toss them. Exception: classic, designer shoes in pristine shape.

Cheap Shoes

Particularly in the dressy category, cheap just doesn't cut it. You are far better off buying a few very expensive, very well-made classic dress shoes than you are buying fifteen pairs of inexpensive shoes. Truthfully, this holds true for every category, but there is a place for inexpensive casuals or trendy shoes that will be worn a season or two and then discarded. In general, expensive shoes far outlast cheap shoes; if well cared for, they always look fabulous; they usually fit better and wear more comfortably; *and* they project an image of taste, refinement, and self-worth.

Fashions fade, style is eternal.
Yves Saint Laurent, French couturier

Forgotten Shoes

If you haven't worn them in two years, review the reasons. If buying them was an obvious mistake, toss them. If you still think they're great shoes, slip them on your feet and strut around the room. If they feel great and you can pull three outfits out of your closet that you wear fairly often and that you would definitely wear these shoes with the *very* next time you put on those outfits, you can hold on to them. If you haven't walked out the door in those shoes six months later, they go.

Duds

If they were a clear mistake and don't say a single, positive thing about you, toss them immediately!

Broken Shoes

If they need repairs, and you're not going to take them to the shoe repair shop within two weeks, toss them. Shoes should always be in perfect working order: clean, polished, and ready to wear. (We'll delve into care and maintenance later.)

If discarded shoes are in good condition, please donate them. If you have a number of expensive shoes, it may be worth a trip to the consignment store; otherwise, send them off into the world and let someone who needs a pair of shoes take them off your hands. Consider it social and material recycling. Breathe and release, girls, and think about the benefits: it frees up blocked chi, bolsters positive fashion feng shui, and even scores karma points! Remember what Grandma always said . . . *Out with old, in with the new.*

closet organization

Before you begin adding shoes to your wardrobe, it's wise to reorganize and create a system to accommodate your new purchases, as well as to best maintain your shoes. As a direct result of a jumbled closet, Sharon Berlan, merchandise product director for a men's footwear department in New York City, inadvertently suffered a fashion *faux pas*. Sharon had worked in the shoe industry since 1984, which offered her the enviable ability to literally travel the world, shopping for shoes in every port. Unfortunately, Sharon lived in a tiny, rent-stabilized, New York City apartment that seriously cramped her style. "Although it was a lovely apartment, near Central Park, with a wood-burning fireplace, I shared it with my boyfriend, which meant I had little to no closet space. I could

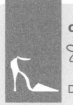

designer dish

Jimmy Choo

DIANA'S DARLING

Jimmy Choo made his first pair of shoes at age eleven and went on to study at London's famous Cordwainers Technical School. Typically, Choo shoes are dainty and seductive, forgoing high fashion and exuding elegance. Even though his shoes are coveted by the rich and famous, and Princess Diana was an adoring patron, Choo describes himself as "a simple man."

never acquire as many personal shoes as I would have liked, and my clothes and shoes were never as organized as I wanted them to be. Far too often they were in a tumbled heap on the closet floor.

"One winter day, before dashing out the door to work, I grabbed a pair of boots from the bottom of the closet. When I arrived at work and began to towel the snow and ice off my boots, I discovered that I had a black leather ankle boot on one leg and a brown leather ankle boot on the other! Even though I had gotten the boot part right, I felt pretty chagrined. As a result, I made the incredibly bold decision to buy a much larger apartment with plenty of closet space!"

Obviously, your imagination and your closet space will determine what you can do, but even a few basics can provide a workable system.

✳ Organize shoes by style (super-sexy sandals, pumps, boots, sneakers, flats, casual, etc).

* To allow leathers to breathe and smells to dissipate, use cardboard boxes or plastic boxes with air holes to store shoes.
* Tape photographs or use a Sharpie to write a description onto the viewing side of the shoe storage boxes. Stack boxes under blouses in the closet or on the closet floor.
* For additional storage, use a shoe/handbag stacker or construct rows of appropriately sized shelving (I like to drape a sexy, see-through curtain over the display to prevent dust accumulation).
* Last, place remaining shoes back in the closet—neatly organized, please.

onward and upward!

Good girl! You've earned a ride in the pumpkin. We'll return to the shoe closet in a few chapters. First we're going to help you refine your image by discussing *shoe attitude* archetypes and how they *strut their stuff*, and then we'll work on specifics in the major categories—work, sex, and athletic footwear. Pour yourself a martini and meet me in the living room!

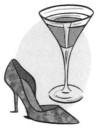

4

defining your shoe personality

Fashion, even anti-fashion, is forever. It's the only way we can become the character we wish to be.

Christian Lacroix, shoe designer

visiting the strutting hall of fame

In this chapter, we're going to explore the Strutting Hall of Fame, where we'll discuss fashion archetypes as a way to define, refine, and expand your fashion personality. What is the Strutting Hall of Fame? Consider it a living museum of *shoe attitude*. Socialites, business leaders, movie stars, television stars, rock stars, and celebrities who cultivated images we love to re-create line the halls. In the interest of helping you develop your individual style, we'll delineate specific categories and introduce the Strutting Hall of Fame members for each: who they are, what they love, how they dress, their habits, and, most important, their *shoe attitude*.

Statistics have shown that 85 percent of the urban population adopts whatever trends they see depicted on television. In today's world, the omnipresent media bombards us with regular reports on socialites and celebrities.

In the early days of Hollywood, when television wasn't available to the masses, radio broadcasts of Oscar ceremonies included descriptions of what the stars were wearing, giving voice to our

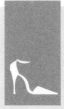

designer dish

Edith Head (1903–1981)

THE ULTIMATE GLAMOUR QUEEN

Internationally known film costume designer; authored The Dress Doctor *and* How to Dress for Success; *one of the first women to lead a design department at a major studio (Paramount)*

Eight-time Academy Award–winning costume designer (nominated thirty-two times), Edith Head believed that clothes told a story about who you were in the world. When designing for top movie stars, including Bette Davis, Marlene Dietrich, Mae West, Audrey Hepburn, Hedy Lamarr, Ginger Rogers, Claudette Colbert, Elizabeth Taylor, Grace Kelly, and many others, Head used what she called "a visual manifestation." She viewed wardrobes as if they were going to be in a silent film to see if you could interpret the characters based on their clothing. Head would also review designs with the actresses, asking them if they felt that the costumes would allow them to more fully transform themselves into the character. "There was magic power in clothes," Head explained. "I could make anyone glamorous."

fantasies and our fascination, and birthing a national obsession. Today, billions of people throughout the world watch the world's best-dressed crowd parade the red carpet, noticing, of course, what dress, what shoes, what hairstyle, and what jewelry Nicole Kidman, Charlize Theron, Jennifer Anniston, and Susan Sarandon are wearing. The next day, we're all trying to emulate them—or at the very least, their *shoe attitude*.

While most of us cannot afford the couturier designs we see these media darlings wearing, we find our own ways to reinterpret their unusual and ambitious ideas. It's important to note that most movie stars are not inherently glamorous; they employ a battalion of stylists to cultivate an image to appeal to their audience. You may have to become your own stylist, but you certainly can learn the tricks of the trade and cultivate the image(s) you'd like to project.

Throughout this journey, you'll serve as your very own shoe mentor—the Fairy Godmother of Shoes—searching for the perfect golden slipper. Where do you look? In the Strutting Hall of Fame, of course! Since most of us are women in search of a solidified fashion identity, you can begin by familiarizing yourself with these examples, searching—in some sense—for your fashion archetype. Will you live your life developing fashion footwear chutzpah, reveling in bombshell mania, or resting comfortably in classic haven?

Keep in mind, these are merely guidelines meant to generate ideas about who you are versus who you would like to be. Some archetypes are more pervasive and deeply ingrained—classics, contemporary classics, femme fatales—others are fringe categories, spinoffs worth mentioning because they possess a distinct style.

You probably will identify strongly with one or two categories, but you may aspire to three or four, at least for certain occasions.

Either way, the women in the Strutting Hall of Fame will help you home in on your existing or desired image and move toward an enhancing cohesiveness. Some may generate ideas for loosening up and inspire you to explore radically new possibilities. Remember, you can absolutely create as many images as you want—one for work, one for play, one for shock value, one for aspiration, one strictly for romance, and so on to the ends of your imagination.

Each category includes classic examples, a brief exploration of the attitude that drives the category, and glimpses into the members' fashion preferences. Okay, let's dish . . . .

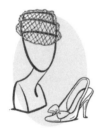

Classic Fashion Icon

Jackie Onassis made luxury frivolity and European glamour de rigueur.

Marie Brenner, author of <u>Great Dames:</u>
<u>What I Learned from Older Women</u>

Den mother: Coco Chanel

Signature shoe: Chanel slingbacks

Favorite shoe designers: Chanel, Gucci, Ferragamo, Louis Vuitton, Yves Saint Laurent, Delman

Inspirational clothing designers: Chanel, Yves Saint Laurent, Valentino, Hubert de Givenchy, Bill Blass, Oscar de la Renta, Christian Dior, Carolina Herrera

Hall of Fame: Audrey Hepburn, Grace Kelly, Jackie Kennedy Onassis, Princess Diana, Carolina Herrera, Queen Rania of Jordan

Shops: Couturier shows, personal shoppers, Fifth Avenue, Bergdorf's, exclusive, expensive boutiques

Classic Fashion Icons believe in elegance; to them, chic means leaving well enough alone. Their most valuable assets: bones, grace, and money. These are women of elegance who radiate authority, know how to gather and maintain substantial social ammunition, always make a good impression without the fireworks, meet every occasion in the proper attire, believe in nonchalant austerity, self-monitor their fashion habits, and disdain trashy fads. This is the afternoon tea crowd, always well-dressed women who rarely make a fashion *faux pas*.

A woman dressed by Coco Chanel in the 1920s and '30s—like a woman dressed by Balenciaga in the 1950s and '60s—walked into a room and had a dignity, an authority, a thing beyond questioning of taste.

Diana Vreeland

Classic Fashion Icons are women who create a distinctive, elegant image. They're the girls born into high society, or at least the girls who studied girls born into high society. They stand tall, shoulders back, and walk slowly. Their makeup is subdued, their hair coiffed, their accessories matched. They adore pale lipstick and prefer their pearls understated—teardrop earrings, chokers, and strands.

They avoid trends like the plague; instead, they wear subdued, refined, high-quality, classic clothing and footwear, but they wear it so well that they develop identifiable, enviable, and highly copied style, eventually winning legendary status, as in "she's so Jackie Kennedy," or "she's got that Grace Kelly thing going on."

In the Strutting Hall of Fame: Audrey Hepburn in Givenchy dresses paired with ballet flats and Sabrina heels, emitting the image of prim perfection. Grace Kelly in the uncluttered, Parisian, $4,000 blue champagne-silk gown she wore to the 1955 Oscars, paired with pearls and long white gloves, immortalizing her fashion icon status. To amp up their drama, these women changed glove length and the size of their pearls.

designer dish

Coco Chanel

CLASSIC ARBITER OF STYLE

Although she had humble beginnings, living in an orphanage from the age of twelve, Coco Chanel transcended her circumstances and created the fashion blueprint for the twentieth century. With the financial backing of two wealthy lovers, Coco opened a millinery business in Paris. Three years later, she opened a dress shop and created a line of casual ready-to-wear, becoming the pioneer of sportswear. Fond of raiding her lovers' closets, she designed satin pajamas and pared-down suits for women, revolutionizing fashion. She created the classic Chanel slingback, the little black dress, and skirt and sweater sets, and popularized short hemlines. Her timeless styles remain popular; for more than eighty years, a woman wearing a Chanel suit, Chanel pumps, and carrying a Chanel handbag always radiated elegance and class. Coco worked relentlessly to create the legendary House of Chanel and was the first designer to release perfume named for its designer (Chanel No. 5).

The Duke of Westminster at one time was madly in love with Chanel. When he asked her to marry him, however, she refused, saying "There have already been three Duchesses of Westminster, but there would always be just one Coco Chanel."

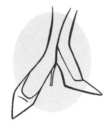

Contemporary Classics

If your clothes wear you, it isn't modern. I'm after much more subtlety. I want the woman and her personality, her own eccentricity, and her own sense of self to come through.

Vera Wang, designer

Den mother: Diana Vreeland

Signature shoe: Sexy high-heeled pumps

Favorite shoe designers: Manolo Blahnik, Jimmy Choo, Christian Louboutin, Salvatore Ferragamo, Stuart Weitzman, YSL Rive Gauche, vintage Christian Dior, vintage Roger Vivier

Inspirational clothing designers: Vera Wang, Tom Ford, Valentino, Armani, Calvin Klein, Chanel, Atelier Versace, Emanuel Ungaro, Oscar de la Renta, Carolina Herrera

Hall of Fame: Socialites CZ Guest and Nan Kempner, fashion editor Anna Wintour, Gwyneth Paltrow, Jennifer Anniston, Nicole Kidman, Catherine Zeta-Jones, Cate Blanchett, Oprah Winfrey, Jane Lauder, Aerin Lauder Zinterhofer, Alexandra Von Furstenberg, Pia Getty

Shops: Couturier shows; personal shoppers to peruse Beverly Hills, Madison Avenue, Bergdorf's, Saks, Neiman Marcus, and exclusive, expensive boutiques

Contemporary Classics are extroverted classics, women who adore elegance yet desire a more contemporary profile. They are extremely efficient shoppers, unafraid to buy multiples of favorites. They love top-grade materials, excellent workmanship, and strong, innovative styling, but shy away from anything over the top. They fall in love with certain designers, but are always on the lookout for

vintage vreeland witticisms

"Unpolished shoes are the end of civilization."

"I loathe narcissism, but I approve of vanity."

"Elegance is important, courage and dignity essential."

[About remaining in Paris during WWII] "Nothing was frightening to me . . . it was all part of my métier, my adventure."

"People should have the taste and talent and use their originality to create a rare ambiance in their daily lives and surroundings."

"The energy of imagination, deliberation and invention, which fall into a natural rhythm totally one's own, maintained by innate discipline and a keen sense of pleasure—these are the ingredients of style. And all who have it share one thing—originality."

someone new; they're willing to experiment as long as the design remains tastefully elegant.

They covet style pizzazz. They are well-rounded, supremely confident, worldly women who refuse to look dated and know the value of adding a few well-chosen trends to spice up their wardrobes. Best described as au courant, they make a major commitment to style and are willing to spend vast quantities of time planning, shopping, coordinating, and executing their wardrobes. Accessories, particularly designer shoes and handbags, are their indulgence.

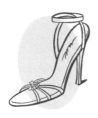

Styling Babe

My name is Sarah Jessica Parker, and I own well over 100 pairs of Manolo Blahniks. I'm not proud of my habit, but it's what I do with my disposable income.

Sarah Jessica Parker

Den mother: Carrie Bradshaw (**Sex and the City** heroine)
Signature shoe: Sky-high, thinly strapped, rhinestone sandals
Favorite shoe designers: Manolo Blahnik, Jimmy Choo, Louis Vuitton, Versus, Sigerson Morrison, Moschino, Roberto Cavalli
Inspirational clothing designers: Marc Jacobs, Prada, Dolce & Gabbana, Giorgio Armani, vintage Christian Dior, Karl Lagerfeld, Stella McCartney, Versace, YSL Rive Gauche, Louis Vuitton, Badgley Mischka
Hall of Fame: Madonna (in real life), Sarah Jessica Parker, Reese Witherspoon, Stella McCartney, Renee Zellweger, Selma Blair (Zappa), Jewel, Jennifer Connelly, Scarlett Johansson, Mischa Barton
Shops: Barneys, Henri Bendel's, Rodeo Drive, Madison Avenue

Styling Babes are Contemporary Classics who maximize and advertise their bona fide sex appeal. They are willing to do whatever it takes to be trendy, hot, man magnets. They love traditional designer labels but are always scouting for hot new talent so they can be the first on their block to have *the* shoes, *the* handbag, *the* leather jacket, and *the* bracelet of the moment. These items become must-haves, and Styling Babes are quick to share the news through public exhibition. They're willing to spend on hot trends and are notoriously fickle. Basically, they're thin girls (thinness being a state of mind) with fat wardrobe budgets. These are the pretty, popular girls of summer.

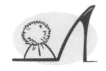

Vivacious Vixen

No doll in the toy box is less played with than Ken. That's because Barbie's relationships are only secondary to her sense of style . . . . Barbie is meant to be fiddled with, thought about, manipulated, done to. All of this aids in a girl making up her mind about who she is and what she wants. That Barbie is a genius.

Jane Smiley, novelist

Den mothers: Barbie, Bond Girls

Signature shoe: Red stiletto pumps worn with everything

Favorite shoe designers: Hollywould, Gianni Versace, Giuseppe Zanotti, Christian Lacroix, Sigerson Morrison, Moschino

Inspirational clothing designers: Prada, Versace, Gaultier, Dolce & Gabbana, DKNY, Michael Kors, Céline, Narciso Rodriguez

Hall of Fame: Brigitte Bardot, Donatella Versace, Heather Graham, Cameron Diaz, Drew Barrymore, Lucy Liu, Jessica Simpson

Shops: Barneys, Bloomingdale's, Fred Segal, West Hollywood, Greenwich Village, European boutiques

A Vivacious Vixen is a Contemporary Classic with sass. Although perceived as ditzy dynamos, they frequently are more clever and bodacious than their peers. They set their own style rules and then gleefully break them, projecting admirable *shoe attitude.* These girls love glitzy glam for dress-up, yet they're not afraid to play in the sandbox. They're experienced shoppers who know and love their labels. Basically, they're the girls who were born gorgeous and learned the value of using their good looks and forceful personalities to get their way. Somewhere between

celluloid dreams: sexy shoes and the movies

The ruby slippers in *The Wizard of Oz*—in a class of their own!

Female Classics

Joan Crawford's and Bette Davis's bitchy 1940s platform shoes

Katharine Hepburn's daringly masculine shoes paired with trousers

Audrey Hepburn's dainty, pointed-toe, princess-heeled pumps

Katherine Hepburn's and Grace Kelly's sleek riding boots

Carmen Miranda's outrageously campy shoes, festooned with fake fruit

Unforgettable Images

Marilyn Monroe's ostrich-feathered mules in *The Seven Year Itch*

Elizabeth Taylor's curling-toed, brocade mules in *Cleopatra*

Jane Fonda's Giulio Coltellacci black-and-silver boots in *Barbarella*

Sophia Loren's stiletto sandals in *Houseboat*

Jodi Foster's bodacious platform shoes in *Taxi Driver*

Julia Roberts's thigh-high, black patent hooker boots in *Pretty Woman*

Whitney Houston's rhinestone platform boots in *The Bodyguard*

All three Charlie's Angels in their *kick-ass* boots!

Femme Fatale and Contemporary Classics, they know how to play up their assets, and they really don't care what other women think. Reportedly, Coco Chanel once offered to give the barefooted, sex-kitten Brigitte Bardot lessons in elegance; Bardot famously rebuffed her.

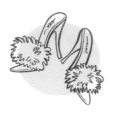

Femme Fatale

People think I am as shallow and superficial as I look, and it's a surprise when they find out, sure enough I am.

Dolly Parton

Den mothers: Mata Hari, Salome

Signature shoe: Stiletto-heeled, mink mules

Favorite shoe designers: Manolo Blahnik, Christian Louboutin, Charles Jourdan, Bruno Frisoni, Versus, Sergio Rossi

Inspirational clothing designers: Elsa Schiaparelli (the anti-Chanel), vintage Oscar de la Renta, vintage Christian Dior, Fendi (furs!), Vivienne Westwood (naughty!), Giorgio Armani (sleek), Dior by John Galliano, Alessandro Dell'Acqua

Hall of Fame: Mae West, Elizabeth Taylor, Sophia Loren, Marilyn Monroe, Jayne Mansfield, Rita Hayworth, Ava Gardner, Dolly Parton, Carmen Electra, Pamela Anderson, Anna Nicole Smith, Paris Hilton

Shops: Expensive lingerie shops

The Femme Fatale, bombshell extraordinaire, really loves dresses, dresses, dresses—curvaceous, sexy, strapless dresses, plunging neckline dresses, defined-waist dresses, pencil-skirted dresses that hug the hips, flowing-skirted dresses that emphasize the curves. The ultimate sex kitten, she's a slinky, seductive siren who likes to wear her hair long, her breasts up, her clothing scanty and tight, and her shoes high.

Femme Fatales seem born to titillate men. Not only are they blessed with natural physical assets, they possess a potent, purring sensuality. These aren't girdle women; their sexy, voluptuous figures are always bursting out of their halter tops and straining the seams of their pencil skirts. They maximize their assets by pampering themselves often—manicures, pedicures, hot oil treatments, facials, breast enlargements, and tons of makeup. They think, act, dress, and breathe sexy. They're anti-chic, preferring instead to slink into a room, looking deadly sexual, turning male heads.

They know the value of showing skin, feminine skin, and their shoe choices are no exception—mules, slingbacks, and thinly strapped sandals, even in winter. They also adore fur coats, diamond tiaras, huge diamond brooches, 5-carat diamond drop earrings, necklaces dripping in diamonds, oversized diamond rings, heavy eyeliner, and big, preferably coiffed hair. Femme Fatales are so popular—and enigmatic—that a series of bombshell books plumb their personalities, tastes, and habits.

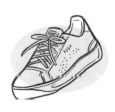

Young Bohemian (Boho)

I don't buy a lot of basics. When I shop for black pants, I'm likely to come home with a scarf and pink shoes.

Kate Spade, designer

Den mother: Ali McGraw

Signature shoe: Vintage Puma sneakers

Favorite shoe designers: Etro, Moschino Cheap & Chic, Miu Miu by Prada, Patrick Cox, Roger Vivier (current), BCBG Max Azria

Inspirational clothing designers: Chloé, Marc Jacobs, Kate Spade, Alexander McQueen, Yohji Yamamoto, Tommy Hilfiger, Badgley Mischka, Baby Phat, Blugirl Blumarine, Zac Posen

Hall of Fame: Kate Spade, Kate Moss, Kate Hudson, Sofia Coppola, Chloë Sevigny, Sheryl Crow, Kate Winslet, Natalie Portman, Claire Danes, Sienna Miller

Shops: Fred Segal, vintage couturier, vintage and modern hippie boutiques, tony thrift shops

Young Bohemians (Bohos for short) have wild, whimsical, eclectic taste, blending couturier with cheap, hippie chic in a way that allows their own quirky personality to shine through. They frequently have bohemian parents whose liberal, creative households encouraged artistic expression and created fashion renegades. Boho girls mix couturier with cheap chic or vintage scores in unique ways, creating a style that ranges between indie glam for dress-up occasions and hippie chic when casual. Actress Sienna Miller, for example, claimed both Audrey Hepburn and Janis Joplin as inspirational fashion icons.

Actress Kate Hudson epitomizes the Young Bohemian. Her free-spirited effervescence pervades all aspects of her life. She exudes a one-of-a-kind, unpretentious, fun-loving, young, experimental, and confident personality that she expresses by mixing and matching designers at whim, occasionally pairing a chiffon Chloé top with torn jeans and a pair of staggering Miu Miu sandals.

Bohos love labels, but they put their own twist on how they wear the labels and set their own standards of acceptability. They adore antique lace and vintage clothing and silk lingerie, often wearing sexy, vintage bustiers and peignoirs as outerwear. They also love recycled furs, original Pucci, and leather in unusual colors. They usually own at least one original Gucci, Prada, Fendi, or Bottega Veneta handbag that they don't hesitate to pair with Marc

Jacobs shoes one day and a funky pair of Target shoes the next. With Bohos, it's all about experimentation, finding your own way, having fun with fashion, and, ultimately, expressing yourself. As Kate Winslet once crowed on the Oprah Winfrey show, "I don't care what people say about my weight . . . I'm just going to hold my head high and be who I am."

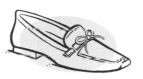

Manly Menace

I always believe that for a woman in a flat shoe, it's up to her to make it really work. Bardot wore ballerina shoes and wonderfully sexy she was. All these girls in the past, like Miss Hepburn, [they wore] just flat shoes, and they really were soooo sexy and feminine.

Manolo Blahnik

Den mother: Amelia Earhart
Signature shoe: Gucci loafers
Favorite shoe designers: Gucci, Ralph Lauren, Hermès, Via Spiga, Tod's, Coach, Bally
Inspirational clothing designers: Ralph Lauren, Calvin Klein, Giorgio Armani, Gianfranco Ferré, Hugo Boss
Hall of Fame: Katherine Hepburn, Marlene Dietrich, Grace Jones, Annie Lennox, Glenn Close; Angelina Jolie and Charlize Theron when they wear tuxedos
Shops: Equestrian shops, menswear departments

Manly Menaces are devastatingly sexy women who adore men *and* the clothes they wear. These are strong women who know that wearing pants can effectively disarm the opposite sex, as well as

shoe attitude on the silver screen

Must-See Classics for Awakening Shoe Attitude

Sabrina (original)

Audrey Hepburn plays an elfin servant daughter, shipped off to Paris, who transforms herself into a sophisticated femme fatale and returns home to steal Humphrey Bogart's heart. Hubert de Givenchy's dresses and Edith Head's overall design savvy created Audrey Hepburn's mystique. This Cinderella story marked the first appearance of Sabrina (kitten) heels, and capri pants paired with ballet flats.

Breakfast at Tiffany's

Features the unforgettable Holly Golightly, a hillbilly Cinderella who transforms herself into a Manhattan playgirl, immortalizing long black evening gloves and cigarette holders in the process. *The* primer on the little black dress, pearls, and kitten heels, in classic Hubert de Givenchy clothes that champion simple and sophisticated elegance.

1980s Favorites

Flashdance

Cinderella goes to dance school! A Pittsburgh steelworker by day and flash dancer by night breaks all the rules by wearing a backless tux, sucking lobster in front of boyfriend, and removing her bra (on a first date!) without removing her seductively altered sweatshirt. She wins the heart of her socialite boss, wins a dance scholarship to Juilliard, and made torn sweatshirts and leggings all the rage.

Desperately Seeking Susan

A wild girl inspires a Jersey housewife to dump her boring husband and hook up with Aidan Quinn. Madonna's jean jacket, parachute pants, fingerless gloves, black rubber bracelets, and wacky, original style created a generation of wannabes.

Pretty in Pink

Adorable Molly Ringwald plays a girl from the wrong side of the tracks who stays true to her own creative bohemian personality by employing clever designs to overcome fashion limitations. Our heroine creates her own ball gown (and her own destiny) when she overcomes her social class to win the (very rich) man of her dreams at the senior prom

Modern-Day Models

Pretty Woman

Cinderella is a hooker in thigh-high, black patent boots held together by a safety pin! Prince Charming plays the part of this Cinderella's Fairy Godmother, transforming her wardrobe and her life, and offering her—in the end—a fairy-tale ending. Please note: our heroine rose to the challenge, boldly stepped into her new shoes, and held out until Richard Gere climbed the fire escape with flowers in his teeth.

Clueless

A trendy, fashion-obsessed, spoiled rich girl comes of age. Alicia Silverstone captures fashionista attitude, replete with an automated closet, computer clothes-matching system, and the ability to pepper conversations with endless, insider fashion references.

Legally Blonde

A seemingly ditzy blonde discovers she's brilliant and dazzles Harvard law school. If you love pink, this one's for you! Reese Witherspoon proves you can be smart and perfectly coordinated, right down to your fashion-conscious Chihuahua.

turn them on. They are usually stalwart, strong-minded, independent women who are who they are and aren't afraid to reflect it in their demeanor, their beliefs, and their fashion. They are frequently athletic, competitive, confident, and victorious. They adore menswear shirts and trousers, paired with oxfords, loafers, and boots.

When Marlene Dietrich first hit the silver screen, Diana Vreeland, the doyenne of American fashion, called her "a fat hausfrau." Paramount Studios costume designer Travis Banton focused on the famous Dietrich legs and either highlighted them by baring them or clothed them in man-tailored suits, successfully creating a Dietrich mystique and transforming her into a glamour queen. Thanks to Banton, Dietrich progressed from "fat hausfrau" to a svelte symbol of style.

Katherine Hepburn epitomized the Manly Menace—in the 1940s!—bravely donning and beautifully wearing Givenchy menswear paired with loafers, and glamorous sportswear paired with tennis shoes. Later, Annie Lennox, another Manly Menace, virtually cross-dressed and still exuded magnetic femininity.

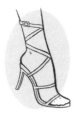

Warrior Goddess
If you've got them by the balls, their hearts and minds will follow.

John Wayne

Den mothers: Joan of Arc, Cleopatra
Signature shoe: Over-the-thigh, skintight boots festooned with buckles and zippers
Favorite shoe designers: Bottega Veneta, Casadei, Guido Pasquali, Bruno Magli

Inspirational clothing designers: Vivienne Westwood, Helmut Lang, Azzedine Alaia

Hall of Fame: Raquel Welch, Barbarella, Emma Peel (<u>The Avengers</u>), Venus and Serena Williams, Anna Kournikova, Angela Bassett, Naomi Campbell; Angelina Jolie, Uma Thurman, and Jennifer Garner when they play superheroes

Shops: Italy for boots; Nike for sport

It all began with Joan of Arc, a teenager so stalwart in her determination she took on kings. Interesting to note that Joan of Arc's refusal to dress in women's clothes was the *coup de grace*; when she resolutely refused to surrender her warrior clothing, they finally sentenced her to death.

Warrior Goddesses work out and love to show off their muscular, bare arms and sexy figures. Impassioned crusaders whose competitive spirits rally around causes, they adopt a take-no-prisoners attitude in everything they do. Like warriors of the past, they relish the feel of leather against their skin—leather shirts, vests, jackets, pants, skirts, even underwear. Their footwear is sturdy, substantial, and intimidating—suede, leather, snakeskin, or crocodile boots with multiple buckles, boots that lace tightly up the leg, or boots sporting animal fur. Gladiator sandals and snakeskin sandals that wind around their legs also bolster their power.

On-screen star Warrior Goddesses date back to Elizabeth Taylor in *Cleopatra*, Jane Fonda in *Barbarella*, and Diana Rigg in *The Avengers* (loved those black leather jumpsuits and black leather boots). Some modern-day Warrior Goddesses include Serena Williams, who believes in shattering records on and off the court and Angelina Jolie, who epitomizes the archetype by donning leg-gripping leather boots and whipping any bad boys who get in her way.

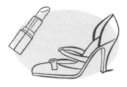

Crafty Coquette

A woman's power lies in coquetry.

Vivienne Westwood, designer

Den mother: Scarlett O'Hara
Signature shoe: Vintage-inspired, brocade pumps
Favorite shoe designers: Emma Hope, Roberto Cavalli, Prada, Sonia Rykiel, Etro
Favorite clothing designers: Badgley Mischka, Cynthia Rowley, Prada, Dolce & Gabanna, Etro, vintage couturier
Hall of Fame: Stevie Nicks, Gwen Stefani
Shops: Small boutiques, vintage stores

Crafty Coquettes are women who learned to be extraordinarily clever. While many are extremely attractive, they are also divinely romantic and gutsy. They forge their own identities and defy anyone to challenge them. They improvise when necessary; think of Scarlett ripping down the green velvet curtains when she didn't have a thing to wear and simply had to impress Rhett to win her way.

The Crafty Coquette possesses southern gentility laced with feminine wiles. She prefers suggestive, flirtatious, feminine clothing and footwear. Her outfits are occasionally overdone, yet infinitely impressive and memorable. She's instantly recognizable, individual, decidedly feminine, and maybe a little intimidating.

In the days of rhinestone 1980s rock-star excess, Stevie Nicks created a gypsy-fairy-sorceress style that made her a standout. By donning predominantly black, ultra-feminine dresses or swirling skirts topped with lacy, sexy bustiers, Stevie won legions of fans by fancifully twirling on stage.

A decade later, Gwen Stefani went from being yet another punkish rock star to the self-created persona of a 1940s-era, platinum blonde, Hollywood starlet, catapulting her to rock-star icon status. Stefani is such a coquette, she created her own clothing line.

To achieve their look, coquettes need coordinating, distinctive accessories: Scarlett had her bonnets, gloves, and umbrella; Stevie had her lace-fringed scarves, brimmed hats, and lace gloves; Gwen had her platform shoes, paste-on bindis, jeweled hair accessories, and bright red lipstick.

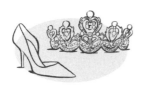

Diva

I never keep anything beautiful in the closet. Even the shoes hang on the wall. Like my Vivienne Westwood dresses from years ago—they are hanging up. I really like to see the beautiful stuff out.

Betsey Johnson, designer

Den mother: Josephine Baker

Signature shoe: High-heeled, sexy, bejeweled sandals

Favorite shoe designers: Christian Dior, Stuart Weitzman, Roberto Cavalli, Sergio Rossi

Inspirational clothing designers: Bob Mackie, Blumarine, Michael Kors, Chloé Boutique, Elie Saab

Hall of Fame: Diana Ross, Aretha Franklin, Tina Turner, Cher, Patti Labelle, Celine Dion, Jennifer Lopez, Beyoncé, Halle Berry

Shops: Couturier shows, Fendi, Rodeo Drive, Las Vegas

Divas are women who marshaled their considerable talent, developed whatever chutzpah it required, and fought their way to the top of the heap. No surprise that they become firmly entrenched in and enchanted with their own image—they're beyond magnificent! They're also not surrendering an inch . . . and why should they? These ladies have earned their lavish lifestyles, outrageous wardrobes, diamonds, and designer shoes. They know who they are, what they love, what they want, and they are used to getting it all, minus any apologies.

Divas make a major investment in how the world perceives them and work hard to maintain their diva status. They've created superstar images, making them the *ultimate* ultimate. They love everything in excess; they love to make a grand entrance; and they require adulation. Their *shoe attitude* says, "Oh yeah, baby, I'm truly fabulous, and aren't you just dying that you're not me?"

Beyoncé and Jennifer Lopez rapidly entered diva status: both adore diamonds, furs, and luxury fabrics so much they each created their own clothing line.

 shoe do

Whose style do you most admire? It may be a celebrity discussed in this chapter or it may be a friend. Whomever it is, darlings, do write down all your observations about the woman you admire and why. In all likelihood, her whole countenance, including her manner of dress, has forged your favorable impression. Now, dream forward and write down ways you can begin to add a little of her magic to your everyday life. *Hint:* Think shoes!

Everyone harbors a little Diva energy. Even if you can only unmask your Diva at costume parties, at least let the poor girl out of the jar occasionally. I promise you that you'll never have a better time.

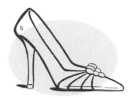

Rocker Chic

No one who was anyone took a handbag to Woodstock.

Carmel Allen, author of <u>The Handbag to Have and to Hold</u>

Den mother: Janis Joplin

Signature shoes: Python boots

Favorite shoe designers: Moschino, Versace boots, Miu Miu by Prada

Inspirational clothing designers: BCBG Max Azria, Prada, Gaultier, Dolce & Gabbana, Baby Phat, Helmut Lang

Hall of Fame: Madonna (on stage), Courtney Love, Lisa Marie Presley, Christina Aguilera, Avril Lavigne, Shirley Manson of Garbage

Shops: Requires outrageous, custom-made clothing and shoes

These girls live to be center stage. They're rebellious, bold groundbreakers. *Hello, I rock and I can do any damn thing I want to do and get away with it.* Courtney Love, who pushed the envelope on downright trashy in the past, went Versace in her private life; on stage, she still loves to shock, but in a more sedate, heroin-chic way. Rocker Chic women blend sexiness with flash and trash. They'll wear flesh-colored lace slips and 4-inch platforms to the opera; fishnet stockings and stilettos to a PTA meeting; and over-the-thigh boots to church. Unless you're in the rock-star business, it's hard to pull off this look in everyday life, but there's no harm in indulging occasionally by donning a pair of over-the-knee suede boots or sandals that wrap a string of rhinestones up your leg. Rock on!

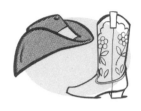

Curvy Cowgirl

I'm the girly-girl of country music . . . I work out so I like to show off my legs . . . There's not a color I won't wear, but pink is my signature . . . I have three pairs of cowboy boots, but they're vintage and wouldn't look out of place in urban hipster circles . . . I wear heels (stilettos) every night on stage.

LeAnn Rimes, singer

Den mother: Annie Oakley
Signature shoe: Vintage cowboy boots or Hermès equestrian boots
Favorite shoe designers: Tony Lama, Hermès, Frye Boots, Ralph Lauren
Inspirational clothing designers: Nudie, Ralph Lauren
Hall of Fame: Shania Twain, Bonnie Raitt, Faith Hill, Wynona, LeAnn Rimes, Shelby Lynne
Shops: Nudie's, Arizona, Nashville, Dallas (Neiman Marcus)

If you grew up watching cowboy movies on television, you might have noticed when, amidst all those dusty, rugged, sexy cowboys, Annie Oakley burst onto the scene wearing fringed skirts and cowboy boots and knocked those boys off their horses. Cowgirls are saucy, vigorous, healthy girls who love to sit in the saddle. Today's cowgirls show a lot more skin and lean more toward tight jeans, but they're still donning those hyper-sexy cowboy boots. If she has all the elements working—suede shirt, rugged jeans, ponytail, and dusty boots—this girl can take casual to the max and look very stylish. East Coast equestrians are high-class cowgirls who can afford a stable of horses, fancy jodhpurs, and Hermès riding boots.

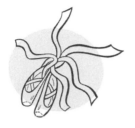

Original

Elsa Schiaparelli slapped Paris. She smacked it. She tortured it. She bewitched it, and it fell madly in love with her.

Yves Saint Laurent, couturier

Den mother: Frida Kahlo
Signature shoe: No such thing!
Favorite shoe designers: Nontraditional, otherwise the gamut; Benoît Méléard
Inspirational clothing designers: Elsa Schiaparelli, Vivienne Westwood, Betsey Johnson
Hall of Fame: Elsa Schiaparelli, Dorothy Parker, Diane Keaton, Bjork, Juliette Lewis
Shops: Vintage shops, eBay, consignment

If these ladies weren't so damn fabulous, you'd be tempted to call their taste bizarre. Originals are multi-textured, creative, eclectic women who sometimes harbor multiple personalities and unabashedly express them. They love to experiment in all areas of their lives; in clothing and shoes, they constantly shake up the mix, *mismatching* color, texture, moods, styles, and price points. They occasionally develop signature pieces, but love surprising everyone, especially themselves. If you're an original, you're always looking for ways to express your individualistic personality, and you're not afraid to break the mold and take the heat.

Dorothy Parker, the wit's wit and the soul of originals, was a plain woman who adored cloche hats so much she made them her signature. If you want to "pull a Parker," you'll have a cloche on your head and a martini in your hand. You might not consider her sexy (although she was frequently so), but you would certainly call her mesmerizing.

After surviving a traumatic car accident in her youth, Frida Kahlo lived and loved full tilt. An original artist and an original woman, she married traditional Mexican clothing with artistic expression. She was a self-possessed, strong woman who developed a style best described as eclectic and unforgettable.

Diane Keaton, our favorite adorable neurotic, also lives life on her terms. Although quite attractive, she seems to go out of her way to hide it. And still, her funky style inspired the wildly popular *Annie Hall* look in the late 1970s and attracted a string of famous lovers. Diane *is* unwaveringly Diane; taking a fashion risk seems as easy to her as brushing her teeth.

the good news

All of the legends and media darlings listed above may have beauty or a certain *je ne sais quoi*, but most begin like you and me—awkward, unsophisticated, and bumbling. In the early days of cinema, when movie studios awarded contracts to upcoming starlets, they signed raw material and then meticulously and deliberately groomed their images. Costume designers—the equivalent of couturier designers— created on-screen and off-screen glamour. Today, most stars hire a team of consultants—costume designers, couturier designers, shoe

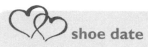 **shoe date**

Choose a movie from the "*Shoe Attitude* on the Silver Screen" lists in this chapter and invite your Fairy Godmother over for a night of indulgence. Pay attention to your heroine's *shoe attitude* and later discuss how it helped her achieve her dreams. Over tea (make it green tea every time you get together, and you'll lose ten pounds by the end of the book!), discuss how you two can incorporate *shoe attitude* into your daily lives. You're starting to feel it, aren't you? How delicious. Enjoy!

designers, and a battalion of hair, makeup, and wardrobe stylists— to cleverly and deliberately construct their images. Most employ stylists to help them select outfits for all important events, thereby enhancing and protecting their desired image.

For those stars who don't rely on professional stylists, the press stands ready to chronicle their fashion blunders. In the early part of her career, Barbra Streisand had difficulty formulating an image. Using the Academy Awards as a barometer, she would show up every year with an entirely, radically different look—a shockingly bad hairstyle and clothing that didn't make sense, let alone make an impressive style statement. Barbra was a fashion-seeking missile, a star in search of an image. These days, she's opted for a refined elegance—rarely changing her hairstyle or her tonal range—because it works. Just ask James Brolin.

Our ultimate goal here is to define and refine your own distinctive *shoe attitude*. When you walk through the Strutting Hall of Fame, which of the outlined archetypes speaks to you? With whom do you most identify—and why? If you could be any of these women, who would you be—at work, at home, in the boardroom, in the bedroom? By reflecting upon the images and attitudes they project and studying how their styles define and empower them, you've taken the first steps toward flushing out your customized *shoe attitude*. You'll be ready to *strut your stuff* in no time. But first, it's time to delve into your sex life to find out whether your *shoe attitude*—or lack thereof—is hindering or helping. Pour yourself a double martini and start thinking about the bedroom!

5

shoes and sex

To me, it's almost like when an actor puts on a costume. It's theatre; it's an act of instant transformation. The woman who buys my shoes [is] exhausted all day, working, and then she puts on the shoes. I'm not a psychoanalyst, [but] I always knew there was an element of desire in shoes. The quick fix is the high heel. It's instant. You put it on and you just have to walk. They make you move differently.

Manolo Blahnik explaining
the attraction of his sexy stilettos

from the moment man invented shoes as a way to protect the feet, woman realized a potent way to titillate her lover, and thus the marriage of shoes and sex began. Does anyone doubt that women who wear high heels are far more likely to have a vital sex life than those who scuff around town in nondescript shoes with minimal sex appeal? In fact, as much as 80 percent of sensory input is visual, and a woman in high heels undeniably delivers potent visual impact. Wearing high heels pitches a woman's body forward, lifts her buttocks 25 percent, arches her back, makes her breasts stand at attention, elongates her calves, and causes her hips to sway seductively when she walks. Those four little *Sex and the City* vixens certainly reaped the rewards of wearing Manolos, Pradas, and Choos all over town.

increasing your sex quotient

When a woman wears high heels, there are only three, real, hopefully insurmountable pitfalls—men, men, men.

Manolo Blahnik, shoe designer

Carrie Bradshaw on *Sex and the City* knew that shoes serve as mood elevators, feminizers, style definers, image makers, sexual enhancers, and wearable art. She loved her shoes—and her shoes loved her right back. Carrie selected shoes to anchor her zany style, a style that defined the way people perceived her and reacted to her. Her shoe choices emboldened her forceful personality and furthered her journey down an artistic, creative, expressive path. Carrie was in bed with her shoes, and when it came to shoes and sex, we all know that girl experienced the double "o" in Manolo. No one had to tell her that anything distinctly feminine excited men or that the mere presence of stiletto heels turned men into Jell-O.

Of course, high heels *are* completely frivolous; in fact, they are blatant evidence that the sexual objectification of women continues. Nevertheless, they are wildly effective, and the truth is we love the way they make us feel, so much so we simply can't help ourselves. Ballet flats, 1-inch heels, and loafers are comfortable and can

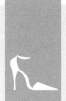

designer dish

Manolo Blahnik

THE DESIGNER'S DESIGNER

Manolo Blahnik is *the* modern master in footwear design. As a child, he watched his mother craft handmade sandals and, discovering a love for fashion, went on to study stage design at the Louvre Art School in Paris. On a trip to New York, Blahnik showed his drawings to Diana Vreeland, and when she saw the shoes he drew on his character's feet, urged him to design shoes. Blahnik studied shoe design and almost immediately began designing and crafting shoes that capture women's imagination and stir lust in their souls. Blahnik creates shoes that epitomize fairy-tale glamour, shoes that women line up to buy. His talent: understanding women. He credits his aunt, who cautioned him about pulling out a woman's chair too quickly. "You must respect the rhythm of her rising from the table," she admonished. Blahnik learned his lessons well; he's dedicated to designing beautiful shoes to help women feel divine. His exceptional eye for line and silhouette, along with his unrivaled craftsmanship, are rare commodities in modern times.

even look sleek, but they're sexually neutral. High heels are impractical, uncomfortable, fragile, anti-utilitarian, overtly feminine, and deadly sexy. A woman in high heels is an instant siren. When you step into the right high heels, a kind of sexual frisson occurs: the tap, tap, tapping of high heels, in concert with the swaying of your hips, combines crackling auditory and potent visual stimulation.

If you want to increase your sex quotient, sexy shoes are the place to begin, and starting at the bottom will quickly bring you to the top of your game. If your closet isn't harboring some sexy stilettos, ultra-feminine mules, slinky slingbacks, glittering rhinestone sandals, drop-dead, calf-hugging boots, or wispy marabou mules, your sex quotient needs a serious boost.

shoe magnetism

Then there is my darling Roger Vivier . . . the shoes he made after he had gone out on his own in Paris are the most beautiful shoes I've ever known . . . shoes made entirely of layers of tulle, shoes of hummingbird feathers, shoes embroidered with tiny black pearls and coral, all with exquisite heels of lacquer . . . a lesson in perfection.

Diana Vreeland, 1984

The attraction of shoes goes beyond purely visual. Shoes can be incredibly romantic. French film star Arielle Dombasle commissioned custom-made shoes to create a fantastic love token. She had a love letter from her husband, along with a lock of his hair and a quill, locked into the see-through heel of a pair of shoes.

In revisiting Cinderella, we find other, more potent, yet extremely delectable associations. For instance, Cinderella's beautiful, precious slipper, into which her tiny foot fit snugly, exercised an unconscious sexual appeal quite beyond the obvious. When viewed as a tiny receptacle into which some part of the body could slip and fit tightly, one could interpret the slipper as a symbol of the vagina, providing a fascinating take on shoe fetishes. In other words, the dainty slipper symbolized what was most desirable in a woman and, thereby, aroused the Prince's male adoration. Although he may not have been conscious of the subliminal vaginal association, when the prince cherished the slipper, he also symbolically expressed his devotion to Cinderella's ultimate femininity.

For the prince, the slipper consciously represented a solution to his quest to find the right bride, one whose femininity would fit his ideal. When he handed Cinderella the slipper, he symbolically validated her femininity. However, referring back to the original Grimm Brothers fantastic rather than fantastical version, it is important to remember that the Prince merely proffered the slipper (*pay attention, my darlings*); and that Cinderella made the empowered choice to remove the wooden shoes of her past and slide her foot into the perfectly fitting slipper of her future.

The fitting of the slipper served as their betrothal. By fitting into the slipper perfectly, Cinderella assured the prince that she had everything she needed; in other words, that everything between them would fit as perfectly as her foot fit into the slipper.

The prince's love for the beautiful slipper (and all that it symbolizes) served as the ultimate male validation of Cinderella's desirable femininity. When he recognized and accepted Cinderella in her degraded state and offered marriage, Cinderella went from borrowed clothing and shoes to owning the real self that had been there all along. Cinderella transformed from a destitute girl who was a shadow of her former self, *forced* to live among the ashes, to a golden princess ready to live her rightful destiny.

At some level, we all replay Cinderella, particularly in the bedroom. We all feel Cinderella magic when we slip our delicate feet into beautiful shoes, and we all expect our princes to swoon. And they do, repeatedly. The real attraction of sexy shoes is that they are so distinctly feminine, and no one understands this basic premise more than a bombshell.

the bombshell shoe philosophy

How to maximize the bombshell in all of us
Hint: all it takes is the right pair of shoes

Sex appeal doesn't depend entirely on physical attributes; it's a kind of vitality and energy—an undercurrent of vitality. It has to do with how you feel as a person.

Dorothy Dandridge, singer and actress

Laren Stover, author of *The Bombshell Manual of Style*, defines a bombshell as "a woman who allows for her frailty and breakable humanity, but does not let it eclipse her aura of glamour . . . a combustible blend of confidence and vulnerability . . . she wears high heels but kicks them off at every opportunity . . . never dresses carelessly and wears marabou mules around the house."

Bombshells have long been misunderstood. In reality, they may be among the smartest women on the planet. They know how to work a room from the moment they strut through the door, and shoes have everything to do with their cachet. Bombshells love flesh-colored shoes that elongate their shapely legs, thinly strapped slingbacks, demure mules, open-toed sandals that show maximum skin, and high heels, even though they infamously remove them as soon as possible. Bombshells adore marabou mules, but only in their boudoirs and only when they match their French lingerie. Unless a particular pair has wickedly pointed toes and 4-inch heels, these women abhor pumps, which they consider far too businesslike for the effect they desire.

So, what's the genius in bombshell wisdom? It's attitude, of course. Bombshells are inherently sexy women who fully inhabit their sex appeal. Every thought, every mannerism, every nuance— hair, makeup, wardrobe, shoes, perfume, even undergarments—and every sashay highlights their sexuality. Bombshells exult in being the most feminine women on the planet, a simple fact they love to flaunt. In doing so, they consistently and gleefully wend hapless men around their stilettos.

Mount on French heels when you go to the ball—
'Tis the fashion to totter and show you can fall.
Eighteenth-century French ditty

For these girls, every day is a dress-up day. They simply do not believe in dressing down. Can you imagine Marilyn Monroe in plain black pumps, Elizabeth Taylor in Keds, or Sophia Loren in rubber thongs? Impossible! Bombshells insist on clothing and shoes that fit their personality and enhance their image. In doing so, they rule the bedroom, which means they're the ones you want to emulate when you want to steam things up. The next time you have an opportunity for a romantic date, pretend you're Sophia Loren in *Houseboat*, or Marilyn Monroe in *Some Like It Hot* or *The Seven Year Itch*, or Elizabeth Taylor in *Cleopatra* or *Cat on a Hot Tin Roof*. Slip on some clingy clothes, tight pencil skirts, sexy, high-heeled mules, and then go out there and growl!

stilettos

High-heeled, thin-strapped sandals have been known to drive some men to frenzies, but . . . they're often men who want to tie you up so be careful.

Cynthia Heimel, humorist, author of <u>Sex Tips for Girls</u>

According to sexologist Alfred Kinsey, a woman who is sexually aroused will arch her feet until they fall in line with the rest of the leg, simulating the position created by wearing unnaturally high heels. Former Gucci designer Tom Ford, when reintroducing stilettos into his collection, cited a similar physiological reason, noting that female baboons walk on tiptoes when sexually aroused. It's small wonder that the French refer to their stilettos as *venez y voir*, or come-hither shoes.

InStyle magazine, exalting their inherent sexuality, once dubbed stilettos "the shoes that launched a thousand fetishes." Considering that stiletto literally means "sharp dagger," it's no surprise that women recognize their ability to weaken a man's resolve. To merely balance in stilettos, a woman must thrust her chest forward and reduce her stride, adopting an undulating sway of the hips that exudes a primal allure.

In *Some Like It Hot*, when Marilyn Monroe sashayed past Tony Curtis and Jack Lemmon in her stilettos, the wiggling and jiggling of her plump bottom made their jaws literally drop. In *The Seven Year Itch*, the vision of Marilyn standing over a grate in a pair of stiletto mules became a classic portrait of sexy 1950s glamour. Marilyn had sensational gams and a bootylicious bottom, and she knew precisely how to flaunt it, on screen and off.

Even though the sixty-plus, devastatingly sexy Tina Turner still dances in them, stilettos are of course impossible to walk any distance in, but they are probably the single most effective shoe a woman can possibly wear. With rare exception, Hollywood stars wear sexy stiletto sandals or mules for important public appearances—although many, quite appropriately, refer to them as limo shoes. Sharon Stone, for example, always looks smashing in her stilettos, but once quipped, "I'm a woman who ends up carrying her shoes."

You don't have to be a movie star to know the value of stilettos. Every woman I know has her own stiletto story. My friend, Terra, an earth mother who feels most comfortable in flat casual sandals, reported that her lover completely surprised her by coming home one night with a pair of outrageous, 5-inch stilettos. "When I put them on, I couldn't even walk across the room in them without falling. Now I only wear them in bed."

Michael Kirby, a manly-man contractor, confided that his wife, Pamela, has a pair of red satin stilettos that always turn him on. "All she has to do is put those shoes on, and my heart starts racing," he said, grinning. "She insists she can't walk in them so rarely wears them, but when I see her pulling them out of the closet, I know it's going to be a sexy night, and I'm perfectly content not to leave the room."

shoe do

Renowned photographer Helmut Newton adored photographing women wearing stiletto heels and nothing else. He thought the form of the stiletto brought out the beauty in the female form. Helmut was right! Ask one of your dearest friends to shoot some erotic, yet tasteful pictures of you wearing stiletto heels and as little clothing as you dare. Bonus points for inventive costuming; extra bonus point for inventive poses!

Jane Endelson Rudes, a teacher in New York City, discovered the power of stilettos. "I was basically a tomboy as a child, which meant I spent the bulk of my childhood in jeans and sneakers. I rarely wore skirts and dresses, and when I did I never considered high-heeled, sexy shoes; I settled for cute ballet flats or fun sandals. As a result, even when dressed to the nines, I felt 'cute' or, at best, 'pretty'—never sexy. I didn't think I cared until a friend talked me into buying a pair of knee-high, brown leather boots with stiletto heels. She convinced me I could wear these boots and suggested I team them with short skirts, tight tops, and funky jewelry to look 'hot.' The first time I slipped those boots on my feet, I felt a surge of energy and stepped out on my date feeling like one of Charlie's Angels. I definitely felt empowered, like I could control and seduce any man I wanted. It wasn't just the sexiness of the stiletto heel; it was the clicking sound they made with every step. I grew to love that sound, so much so I often double-clicked just for fun! When I walked into a room wearing those boots and heard the clicking sound on a hard floor, I felt powerful, almost immortal."

A dress makes no sense unless it inspires a man to want to take it off.

Françoise Sagan, writer

Lorraine Bates, a former cabaret singer in New York, had a pair of black leather, high-heeled, open-toed shoes that she remembers as *raison de etre* to strut. "They became so ingrained with my cabaret act I couldn't envision going on stage without them. When the lights dimmed and the announcer spoke my name, I stepped out from behind the curtain in those shoes, feeling taller than life. I

the fetish behind the fashion

Beginning in the tenth century, upper-class Chinese bound their small daughters' feet to "sculpt" them into the highly desirable shape of lilies, preferably no larger than five inches at adulthood. They referred to a three-inch foot as a "golden lotus," while a four-inch foot was a "silver lotus." Some consider high heels a parody of binding—stiletto heels force women's feet into a similar position, and erotically charged fetishes generated both traditions. In binding, however, slowly unwrapping the lengths of cotton or silk bandages that tightly bound their wives' crippled feet served as foreplay for Chinese men, who sometimes used the bandages to tie their wives to their beds, rebinding the feet after the act.

loved the clicking sound they made as I strutted around the stage, a staccato rhythm that signaled my femininity and infused me with power. My shoes gave me attitude; attitude that carried forth into my act. One of my favorite moments in the act came when I sat on a stool and crossed my legs, flaunting my gorgeous shoes for all to see, baring the sexy ankles and taut calf muscles they created. I wore the shoes without stockings, and the combination of knowing how sexy they made me look, combined with the sensuality of feeling warm leather against my skin, made me feel every inch a woman. Even if exhausted, after most shows, I would dance all night in those high-heeled, sexy shoes."

Evidenced by the proliferation of Web sites and store window displays in major urban areas, where they reign as featured shoes, stilettos hold mass appeal. They have, of course, found a natural home among people with a foot fetish. In the 1980s designer

Vivienne Westwood, along with co-designer Malcolm McLaren, blurred the lines between sex and fashion by creating a selection entitled "Erotic Zones" featuring bondage trousers, peephole pants, masturbation skirts, and a penis shoe. The penis shoe had two oversized puff balls at the top of a stiletto heel, feathery black puffs at the base of the toe, and a black patent penis that curled upward another three inches beyond the toe. That's taking it way over the top, of course; a simple stiletto will suffice. Face it, girls, stilettos basically are the equivalent of sexual dynamite, particularly when they include maximum skin exposure (spaghetti straps or mules), open toes, sexy fabrications, or ankle straps.

for the stiletto-challenged

As much as we wish it weren't true, many of us simply cannot wear stilettos. While they may be the crowning jewels, stilettos are not the be-all-and-end-all of sex appeal. Let's talk options!

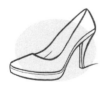

Find a Platform

The fresh, empowering perspective of height

I like to put a woman on a pedestal.

Vivienne Westwood, designer

If stilettos feel too restrictive or taboo for your tastes, platforms are another sexy option. Between rocker chicks and hookers, platforms have a long, somewhat sordid history of sexual innuendo.

They actually date back to fifteenth-century Venice, where fashion-able women adopted a style popularized by prostitutes and tottered around their houses on 10-inch platforms. While historians conjectured that Venetian men may have preferred unwieldy platforms that limited their wives' ability to stray, modern women seem to like the extra height or possibly the sense of power that elevated platforms provide.

My petite friend Stefanie Charren, an event planner and public relations guru, loves her 4-inch platform boots. "Whenever I have a major event, I'll wear whatever outfit works with my platform boots. I need those boots; they give me a kick-ass attitude. No matter how big the event, as soon as I show up in my boots, not only do others seem to instantly respect me, in no time I'm bossing people around and running the whole show with a new level of confidence."

Platforms combined with skintight, over-the-knee boots create a particularly potent sexual charge, and rocker chicks get a lot of mileage out of adding rhinestones or motorcycle buckles, zippers, and chains. Add a pair of fishnet stockings, and you push the sexual quotient even higher.

 killer heels

Vivienne Westwood created the 10-inch elevator platforms that tumbled super-model Naomi Campbell during a fashion show in the early 1990s, the photo-graph of which circulated worldwide.

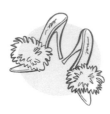

Mules, Mules, Mules

The distinctly feminine art of showing a little skin

People want to look taller and thinner. No one ever says "Ooh! Let me buy that dress because it makes me feel matronly."

Michael Kors, designer

Mules are the bikinis of footwear. The thing that makes them so alluring is not simply the way they bare so much skin, making you look instantly taller and thinner, but the way they so easily slip off the foot. Like stilettos, mules are distinctively feminine footwear. Women's legs look luscious in delicate mules—banded mules in sexy snakeskin or alligator for daytime; sexy satin mules adorned with rhinestones for the evening; marabou or feather-trimmed mules for the boudoir.

On the plus side, low-heeled mules can look pretty sexy, particularly compared to loafers, oxfords, flat sandals, or sneakers. But, if you want to wow men, buy high-heeled mules, and then master the art of slipping them off, or, even better, very seductively dangling them from a carefully crossed leg.

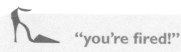

"you're fired!"

Marla Maples, the woman who stole Donald Trump away from Ivana, fired her male publicist when she discovered he was stealing her shoes to fulfill his sexually charged shoe fetish.

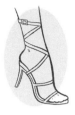

Stiletto Substitutes

Ways to develop a sexy profile and maximize your sex appeal irrespective of heel height

To define feminine only by ruffles, a girdle, high heels, and skirts that must be pulled down all the time is obsolete, like steel corsets and girdles.

André Courrèges, designer

If you want to spice up your sex appeal and you can't wear stilettos or can't afford $400 Manolo Blahnik, Jimmy Choo, or Prada stiletto sandals, you can still dazzle the boys. Buy the sexiest highest-heeled red shoes you can manage and wear them very occasionally and very pointedly, such as when entertaining a lover at home. Casually cross your elongated legs and dangle one shoe provocatively. Or ceremoniously, and suggestively, slip them off. Or wear flats to the restaurant and slip on the heels just before entering the restaurant. Or slip them on with a pair of silk stockings, a garter belt, and little else, and bring your lover a martini. Five minutes should do it.

Many men also find relatively sedate, yet distinctly feminine shoes titillating. I once dated a man who admitted to me that the mere sight of my lipstick on a cup excited him. Imagine what a pair of luscious, merely feminine shoes could do. French shoe designer Christian Louboutin, for example, considers shoes *objets d'art* and has trademarked a red leather sole reminiscent of lipstick to evoke femininity. He also heightened romance by encasing love letters, flower petals, and locks of hair in clear vinyl Lucite heels. If you can't afford Louboutin, a lace-trimmed, brocade pump on a kitten heel can be effectively romantic.

hot buttons

Victorians considered corsetlike high-button shoes coquettish; they emphasized a woman's delicately turned ankle and implied opportunities for lovers to slowly unbutton them during seduction.

Arlene Corsello, a photographer in Sacramento, California, remembered a pair of shoes she bought in the 1960s. "I had very little control over my life at the time and was feeling extremely insecure about my relationship. When shopping one day, I saw a pair of fabulous, black, fake-alligator shoes. They had very, very pointy toes, a sexy, low vamp, a wide buckle, and a relatively short heel that was extremely narrow in the center but literally flared at the bottom. They looked like a pair of glamorized witch shoes, and I had long been fascinated with witches and the magical powers they supposedly possessed. I remember thinking that they just might bring me luck, and they did! As soon as my boyfriend saw me in those shoes, he thought I was hot stuff, which had everything to do with how much I absolutely loved those shoes and felt both bewitchingly feminine and empowered when I wore them."

Slingbacks, which Laren Stover, author of *The Bombshell Manual of Style,* calls the trademark shoe for bombshells, are extremely feminine, elegantly sexual shoes; a barely visible, delicate strap can be extraordinarily sexy on a slender, naked heel. In fact, according to Stover, bombshells believe so strongly in the seductiveness of open shoes and bare legs that they regularly brave freezing temperatures sans stockings in the name of bewitching men.

Strappy, open sandals of any height, particularly when accessorized with a saucy pedicure, delicate toe rings, glittering ankle bracelets, or droplets of perfume snuggled in-between toes can make a man's pulse quicken. Gold Mata Hari snake sandals winding up your leg can be extraordinarily seductive (perhaps they conjure images of Eve squashing the temptress snake in the garden). Ultra-feminine, jewel-studded sandals on any heel height or moderately heeled, delicately strapped goddess sandals paired with flowing, formfitting goddess dresses are divinely sexy, particularly in exotic materials or rhinestones. Silken wraps spiraling up a bare leg, paired with a sexy, silky skirt and plunging decollete or strapless blouse, also are sexy stiletto substitutes. And thong panties aren't the only thongs guaranteed to quicken a man's pulse. Rhinestone thongs, jeweled thongs, snakeskin thongs, red satin thongs, beaded or feathered thongs—on your feet, not your buttocks—can be supremely sexy.

A woman waits motionless until she is wooed. That is how the spider waits for the fly.

George Bernard Shaw

And then there's leather. Whether it makes them feel like cowboys, bomber pilots, or bikers, men love leather—particularly head-to-toe leather. Thigh-high boots that stop just short of your heavenly gate are particularly erotic. Shiny, shin-hugging patent boots, lace-up boots, buckled or zippered boots, and fur boots all are sexually enticing. Wearing a leather corset with a pair of thinly strapped leather sandals that lace up your leg also is pretty alluring. Wearing leather pants or a leather skirt with matching leather boots seems to rev up men's engines. And if you throw in a whip, you're really in business . . . which leads us to the all-important props.

props

The clever use of stockings and garters

We should be dangerous characters. Just think of Garbo and Dietrich and Harlow—they were really dangerous. When they gave a man the come-hither look, the poor guy didn't know whether he was going to be kissed or killed.

Kim Novak, bombshell actress

Reportedly men notice their lover's aura before they notice her clothing or shoes. Personally, I think this happens in a split second, of which the poor dears aren't even conscious. Clever girls can maximize this opportunity, so set the stage, darlings.

 ancient inspiration

Fashion icon and longtime fashion editor Diana Vreeland is credited with inventing the modern thong sandal. As one of the first women permitted to view the bordello district of ancient Pompeii, she spied a drawing of a naked slave, frozen in *flagrante delicto*, wearing a thong sandal. She commissioned a shoemaker to create one for her, and it quickly became her signature casual shoe and a classic casual shoe for millions of grateful women.

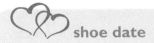 **shoe date**

It's time to leave your Fairy Godmother behind. Mail a perfumed note to your favorite prince inviting him to a night out on the town. Really get into the mood by selecting a sexy dress and daringly sexy shoes. Set the stage, including luxurious perfume and love songs. Don't warn the poor darling; surprise him, and then wallow graciously in his adoration! *Hint*: Be ready for anything, and repeat often.

Obviously, you want to create a seductive environment. When the Duke of Windsor invited Wallis Simpson to join him for their first weekend alone, the financially strapped divorcee threw caution to the wind and spent a small fortune on handmade French nightgowns, so intricate they required three weeks to fashion. Intent on winning the Duke's heart, Ms. Simpson knew her looks weren't enough, and thus hounded the seamstress daily so as to have the precious gowns in time. Ms. Simpson knew the value of staging; by the end of the weekend, the Duke was hers.

Wearing slinky, shiny fabrics, donning red lipstick, and showing a little skin will create a sexy state of mind—for you and for him. Imagine sprinkling sensuality liberally throughout the room. If you don't own pink marabou mules and a matching pink-marabou-trimmed robe, you're missing a serious stage prop. Wearing them is fabulous for creating *shoe attitude*, but simply positioning them in your boudoir or toilette can set the stage for high jinks.

Although it's the shoes, it's not *just* the shoes. Accessorize shamelessly—corsets or lacy garter belts and silk stockings, patterned stockings, fishnet stockings, perfumed oils, tanning lotions, henna tattoos, glitter dust, fabulous nightgowns, and a great attitude. Sure, shoes make a huge difference, but men adore silk stockings and garter belts, and if they're part of your arsenal, he'll be purring at your feet and removing your shoes in short order. Have fun, girls!

outrageous accoutrements

Sexy surprises to spice up your sex life

A woman shod by Roger Vivier who went out stark naked would appear very much dressed.

Yves Saint Laurent

To really rock your lover's world, accessorize your fantasies with these items to wear (or not wear) with your most outrageous pair of shoes:

* Full-length fur coat, bare underneath
* Short fur jacket, racy panties, racy bra
* Fur jacket, garter belt, black stockings, panties optional
* Fringed leather cowgirl jacket
* Black leather motorcycle jacket, and chain-mail ankle bracelet
* Sexy corset, matching stockings
* Lace teddy, garter belt optional
* Sexy garter belt, black or red stockings
* See-through negligee
* Extremely feminine undergarments, handcuffs
* Thong, pasties, glitter
* A truly fabulous hat on your head

* A truly fabulous hat cleverly positioned
* Fabulous sunglasses, a la Jackie O
* A stunning diamond or rhinestone necklace
* A stunning navel ring
* Absolutely nothing

Sex appeal emanates from how you feel when you slip on a pair of shoes that excite you, whether they bring out the beast in you or turn you into a simpering sex kitten. Any shoe that makes you feel sexy, feminine, desirable, and hot will make your partner salivate.

Now that we've outfitted you for the bedroom, it's time to suit you up for the other frontier—the boardroom!

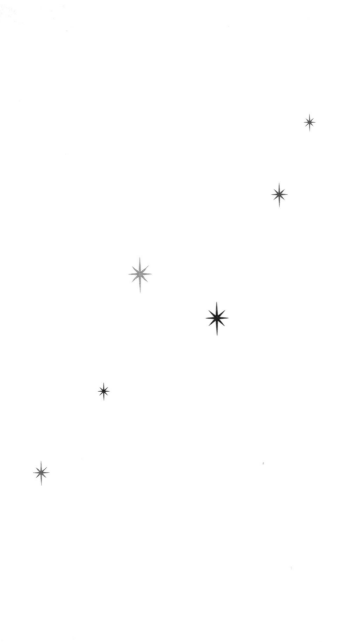

6

up the corporate ladder in high heels

Men do not wear shoes they can't walk in . . . We gals are not going to be able to get to the top in this world if we can't walk there, let alone run . . . Men understand this, their idea of a great shoe is one that feels so good they forget they are wearing it . . . face it, if we say "These boots are made for walkin'," then hobble away, trip over the rug, and fall flat on our face, then how empowering is that?

Susan Jane Gilman, author of <u>Kiss My Tiara</u>

ow that we've amped up your sex quotient, it's time to focus on the importance of image in the workplace. If you want to be a tigress in the workplace, you may need to redefine and refine your corporate or business image. You already know that smart girls go beyond the typical dress for success, so we'll focus on how specific footwear choices empower women in corporate America and how changing from one style to another can literally jump-start your career. Basically, your wardrobe choices reflect your focus, intention, and determination to move up in the world, so if you have been downplaying your corporate savvy, revamping your work wardrobe can instantly revamp your career. How do you get there? First you determine your goals, and then you determine all the necessary steps to get there, including, of course, the requisite image. Then, you work on letting go of old ways of thinking about yourself so you can open up to new ways of thinking, acting, and living.

We all know that the way we look greatly influences our lives; every time we buy new clothes or shoes, we long for our purchases to change our lives and become a magical symbol of confidence. If you're reading this book, you probably already are, or want to be, a trailblazer, someone who sets the pace, leads the way, and moves into new territory confidently. If you've already marched, or are intent upon marching, up the corporate ladder, you well know that blending into the background didn't, or won't, get you there. Instead, you need to think, act, and dress like a rising star in your field.

crafting your corporate image

She was always well-groomed, there was a consequential good taste in the plainness of her clothes, the blues and grays and lack of luster that made her, herself, shine so.

Truman Capote, author of <u>Breakfast at Tiffany's</u>,
describing Holly Golightly

So, here's the big question: Are you in command of your own life? I don't mean do you have a general idea about how your life is

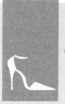

designer dish

Charles Jourdan

BREAKING THE MOLD

In the 1930s, Charles Jourdan became the first shoe designer to advertise his shoes in fashion magazines. In the 1970s, he broke the mold again by creating ads using surreal settings, fantasy shoes, and artistically arranged photographs as a component of a larger story, linking shoes to wit and mystery.

progressing; I mean are you *the* five-star general in charge of your life? It's a simple fact that in order to reach your goals, you first have to define them. By focusing on what it is you want to accomplish or become, and literally writing down your goals in black and white, you invest energy into making them happen. As you gain clarity and create a set of tangible goals, you also develop the persona that accompanies your vision. And then, *girlfriends*, it comes down to this: dressing that persona brings additional, potent energy to manifestation.

I once had a writing teacher who told me to act as if I were already confident, poised, capable, and working as a writer. At the time, my goals centered on generating creativity. Thus, I began by envisioning how an imaginative writer would reflect creativity, originality, and pizzazz, and decided that accessories were the ideal means for inner and outer expression. Shortly thereafter, on a business trip to New York with my husband, I spied a pink suede baseball cap covered with rhinestones in a Trump Tower store. (Rhinestone-studded garments were very popular in the 1980s.)

The hat cost $64, an exorbitant price for me to pay for a frivolous item, so I admired it, but ultimately passed on it. That night, I dreamt I was sitting at my desk finalizing my novel, and that little pink suede baseball cap was clamped tightly on my head. The next day, I rushed back to the store and bought the cap.

When I returned to California, feeling completely inspired, I bought a pair of hot-pink, high-top Converse sneakers and added rhinestones. I even bought a white T-shirt and emblazoned "writer" on its front in rhinestones. I may have looked slightly comical in my getup, but when I put them on, I felt very much an inspired, creative, and imaginative writer. Amazingly, acting (and dressing) as if I were already a successful author helped me manifest the desirable traits—discipline, diligence, thinking outside of the box, being willing to shake things up, and so on. I wore out the sneakers and T-shirt, but, twenty years later, I still have what I affectionately and respectfully call my "creativity cap."

When it came time to become a professional writer promoting herself in the business world, I opted for knee-high, purple suede boots, teamed with a denim pencil skirt and expensive, one-of-a-kind

 exercising your rights

Rapid social and economic change from the mid-1800s forward led to a realization that women could choose the way they wanted to dress. Many women exercised their right to dress as they pleased. In order to be comfortable during protests, women suffragettes wore broad-heeled sensible shoes, which became quite fashionable as a result. According to Linda O'Keeffe, author of *Shoes*, "By the 1920s women's bodies were liberated, and so were their feet."

sweaters. Basically, I wanted my clothing to express my creative originality, as well as present a pulled-together, polished, professional look.

Like most of us, Michelle Cunnah, author of chick lit novels *32AA, Call Waiting,* and *Confessions of a Serial Dater* (a Cinderella story based on her life, no less!), grew up searching for a fashion identity. "I was reading fashion magazines and trying to mold myself into something, and failing rather badly. Finally, I met an older woman at work named Maureen, who took an interest in me. I had just taken a higher-level job and was searching for a way to match my appearance to my ambitions. Luckily, Maureen reflected the epitome of style; even luckier, she and her daughter even wore the same size clothing and shoes as I did! Even though I had the sneaking impression she didn't need to discard anything, she would invite me over to her house for dinner and closet-cleaning sessions. She would recommend clothing and shoes for me, and I would leave with armloads of clothes and shoes infinitely better than the ones I typically wore. Clearly, she was steering me in a certain direction, but she was so clever about it, I never felt belittled; I felt uplifted, inspired, supported, and encouraged. She obviously took great delight in helping me, molding me, if you will, and I was simply thrilled to discover my very own fashion mentor, someone who taught me how to select clothing and shoes that boosted my personality. Without even thinking about it, I gradually absorbed Maureen's style attitudes, and they have served me well."

Ideally, somewhere along the way you'll acquire a fashion mentor, but in the meantime, you can launch your transformation by carefully listing your career goals—and all the necessary steps to get there—including the style of clothing, accessories, and shoes you'll need to become that person. To begin, study the upper ranks of your chosen market. If you want to get to the top, you'll have to aim for the top and dress the part.

It helps to imagine you are an actor preparing for a new role: you're an artist transforming into a pharmacist; edgy and disorganized transforming into cool, calm, and collected; flamboyant transforming into ultra-conservative; an accountant transforming into political humorist; meek transforming into reactionary; constricted transforming into expansive; pastels transforming into brights.

How you dress affects how you feel and how you interact. If you want to dress for success, dress to impress; dress to project the image of a mover and shaker; dress to win positive assessments; dress to create an image of someone who is always reaching for the higher rung. When your boss or your potential clients favorably notice what you are wearing, they tend to remember you as someone with flair. The cumulative effect: Your boss and the client think about you when it comes time to award projects and promotions.

I can't understand how a woman can leave the house without fixing herself up a little, if only out of politeness. And then, you never know, maybe that is the day she had a date with destiny, and it's best to be as pretty as possible for destiny.
Coco Chanel

One of our favorite shoe heroines, Diana Vreeland, used fashion as an instrument for power and prestige—and very successfully so. Ms. Vreeland once noted that her looks were marginal at best, so she used her eye for fashion to create a distinctive image. She was dancing on the roof of the St. Regis Hotel—wearing a white Chanel dress, a bolero, and a rose in her hair—when Carmel Snow, editor of *Harper's Bazaar*, noticed Diana's unique and distinctive style and immediately offered her a job. Vreeland went on to become Editor of *Harper's Bazaar* and *Vogue*, through which she dominated the fashion world for decades.

If Diana can do it, we can do it! To launch your corporate makeover, consider the following series of questions:

* What's your ultimate corporate objective?
* Whose attention are you trying to gain?
* What impression do you want to create?
* Who do you admire, and how do they dress?
* How have you been shortchanging yourself?
* What would be the benefits of making a radical change: self-confidence, self-esteem, and emotional satisfaction?
* Do you look pulled together, polished, professional, and ambitious? Or do you look like you don't really care about the impression you make?
* Do you flounder on either extreme: assertive or passive; feminine or masculine; powerful or safe; individual or bland; creative or boring?

* *And, finally, what's in your shoe portfolio?*

Before we move into a strategy for aiming higher, consider the following absolute basics when creating a positive impression in the corporate world.

* You are always making an entrance. Put as much thought into your outfit as you do your presentation.
* Knowing how to mix and match clothes, shoes, and accessories is the single best way to add cachet to your image.
* The best heel height for professional shoes is 2½ inches, but even 1-inch heels will look more professional than flats.
* Selecting a signature color and style simplifies wardrobe coordination and helps create a distinctive image . . . *it's so you.*

aiming higher

Dressing for the job you want

You can have anything you want in life, if you dress for it.

Edith Head, Oscar-winning costume designer

While the absolute basic tenet for aiming higher in the corporate environment is that appropriate *and* chic sends the message that you *are* going straight to the top, the worst *faux pas* you can make in the corporate environment is being underdressed. Luckily, my mother was a southern lady whose ideas about how a young woman dresses set me on the road to success early. My mother never allowed me to wear jeans to school, and even forbade them for normal teenage events, like trips to town, a night at the movies, or even the local carnival. Of course, as a teenager, these strictures mortified me. I constantly smuggled jeans over to my best friend's house and changed at her house before and after we went anywhere.

However, when I moved to New York City right out of college, my mother's rules served me well. I never questioned the need to wear dresses to work, along with well-groomed shoes. While many

hmmmm

Did you notice in the movie *Working Girl* that top boss and corporate raider Sigourney Weaver always wore high-heeled pumps, while the battalion of secretaries dressed a bit trashy and either wore clunky platform shoes or donned sneakers? Take note: Melanie Griffith stole clothes right out of her boss's closet to successfully masquerade as an executive.

of my colleagues dressed down, I dressed up. And up I went, winning five promotions in seven years. Sure I worked hard, but I also dressed for success. Every time I gained a promotion, I wisely promoted the way I dressed. In other words, I stayed ahead of the game by looking and acting as if I already had the higher job. When it came time for someone to move into those positions, my superiors easily envisioned me as their candidate.

Years later, when I managed a staff of young women, I set dress standards and encouraged them to "dress for the job you want." Particularly these days, when casual wear has infiltrated all aspects of our lives, many of these young women didn't have a clue how to dress up. More than one needed gentle coaching. Because they invariably had very limited budgets, I gave them simple guidelines: two pairs of classic, high-quality black pants; three well-cut, crisp blouses; a sweater set; a black skirt; a classically cut plain dress; a blazer; two pairs of low-heeled, relatively plain pumps; one pair of moderately high heels. This minimal wardrobe always got them started and always impressed the company president.

Obviously, every corporate setting has its own dress codes. Pay attention to what others are wearing, particularly the women who

shoe do

Let's pump up! Seriously, it's time to find a pair of pumps that make your heart thump *and* amp up your corporate image. We're not talking basic black on low heels or chocolate suede on stacked heels; we're talking red, purple, green, or pink suede, fake alligator, or snakeskin on a 3-inch heel that you can pair with your classic suits to punch up your image.

are in the positions you want, and then copy their manner of dressing, adding your individual flair. Begin with a simple wardrobe, but build smartly toward the future you want.

Marcela Landres, an editorial consultant in New York, has used shoes as markers for her professional development. "Like everyone else, in college, I lived in inexpensive sneakers. When I began my professional career, very far down on the food chain, I recognized a need to wear professional shoes. Even though I could barely afford them, I bought and wore Nine West black loafers and boots. When I won my first promotion, to celebrate my victory and remind myself that I was climbing the ladder and needed to look the part, I splurged on a pair of brown Coach loafers ($150). With my second big promotion, I sprung for my first pair of truly fabulous shoes—a pair of Isaac Mizrahi black linen slingbacks with a patent lining and kitten heels ($125 on sale!). By this time, I was convinced that wearing expensive shoes created an aura of professionalism that others saw and I felt."

Up until recently, Marcela selected neutral colors—brown, black, and beige. However, just about the time she won her latest promotion—"where I would never be anyone's assistant again"— she was editing a book entitled *Feng Shui Chic*, a unique guide about using the principles of feng shui on your body, via clothes, accessories, makeup, jewelry, hairstyle, and, of course, shoes. "This book said the color red was good for overall business and particularly potent for strengthening fame and reputation. Since I wanted to raise my industry profile, as well as celebrate my most recent promotion, when I spied a pair of cherry red, Jimmy Choo slingbacks on a kitten heel ($300), I knew they were the perfect shoes for the next phase of my life.

"The first time I wore them, I felt amazingly powerful and unforgettable. I've been wearing them—with a monochromatic outfit, usually black or blue—to public speaking events, and I am always a standout. I've found it almost impossible to feel lackluster in my red Jimmy Choos; they're worth every penny. They definitely helped me feel successful, so much so I've already got my eye on a pair of Manolo Blahniks."

When purchasing your corporate clothing and shoe wardrobe, keep the following suggestions in mind, particularly in light of their subliminal messages.

Quality Before Quantity

Wearing cheap clothing and shoes may send a subliminal message that you don't have an appreciation for quality or that you don't hold out for the best. Buying quality items sends a message that you possess excellent taste *and* wisely delay financial investments until you can afford them. If your boss sees you strategizing the way you buy clothing, he'll deduce that you strategize well in business.

Flattering Before Variety

Displaying a large wardrobe containing many (inexpensive) items that don't fit your age, your status, or your body type will send the message that you have poor assessment skills. Wearing four or five outfits that perfectly fit your age, your status, and your body type sends the message that you know who you are, where you fit in, and how to maximize your assets.

Conservative Before Fashionable

Wearing highly fashionable clothing may send a message that you don't have a clear sense of who you are. Wearing conservative yet individualistic clothing and shoes sends a message that you exert common sense, know who you are, and exercise strong value judgments when making financial decisions.

At some point it will be time for your boss to promote from within. Have you maximized all opportunities to make sure it's you who comes to mind? Getting dressed should remind you that you are more than your current position title; you are headed somewhere. Clothes and shoes lead the way, opening doors into your new life. They help establish inner and outer credibility. Think of it as coaxing yourself into a new life.

no playing it safe

Forging a style all your own

Clothes and courage have much to do with each other.

Sara Jeanette Duncan, first full-time
female journalist at the <u>Toronto Globe</u>

If you're not forging your own fashion identity, you may inadvertently be sending a message that you always play it safe, have little to no personality, lack originality, or don't take necessary risks.

While you don't want coworkers to characterize you as someone who runs all over the fashion map, you do want to take calculated risks. Look for a common, stylistic thread that both reflects your personality and projects your best self, and then weave it into your wardrobe. Maybe you adore pencil skirts and happen to have fabulous legs that mid-heel, snug-fitting suede boots show off effectively? Instead of buying classic brown or black, buy boots in fringe colors like forest green, red, or baby blue suede. Style consistency lends an air of authority; in general, it's best to avoid fads altogether and blend trends into your wardrobe discriminately. Steer away from unfounded experimentation, like sinking $300 into genuine-fur-trimmed ankle boots, and anything with blatant sexual overtones, such as fishnet stockings or 5-inch sculpted-steel stilettos.

Class comes in how you put things together. You can greatly enhance a standout image through the clever use of accessories. Style is what flatters you, what appeals to you, what makes your heart sing, what makes you feel sassy. Show off what you love; keep in mind, however, that anything perceived as razzmatazz—zebra-fur pumps, or mink pompons on ankle boots, for example—deflects from a professional image.

According to Carole Swann Meltzer, feng shui master and author of *Feng Shui Chic*, you can choose particular colors, shapes, and fabrications to enhance certain impressions. For instance, in relation to shoes, she believes you can enhance or attract the following qualities through clever choice in color, fabrication, or shape.

Meltzer recommends open-toed patterned shoes for creativity; square-toed boots for power; red pointed toe high heels or boots for action; beige or brown flats for balance, silver or gold closed-toe slingbacks for wisdom; and my favorite, red shoes for fame!

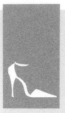

designer dish
Kenneth Cole

GENIUS

Superstar designer Kenneth Cole thought outside of the box when he struck out on his own. In 1982, to launch his brand, Cole rented a 40' trailer, bought a video camera, and set up outside the Fashion Footwear Association of New York show. Cole hired models and security to limit entrance to a few people at a time—implying his line was hot, hot, hot—and sold more than 40,000 pairs of shoes in two days!

You don't need to overthink every choice, but in taking the idea of *Feng Shui Chic* dressing a bit further, Meltzer suggested that it is also possible to create negative connotations based on what you are wearing in the corporate environment. Some examples include:

* Peasant blouses and gypsy skirts paired with thong sandals may make you look like a peasant.
* Loose clothing accessorized with soft, slouchy boots may make you look unstructured.
* Flamboyant clothing and shoes, such as fur coats and $500 leather boots, may make you look like a showoff.
* Sexy clothing and shoes, such as cleavage-revealing blouses and 4-inch stilettos, may make you look like a showgirl.
* Plain, boxy, or tightly contained clothing and plain black lace-up oxfords may make you look like someone who has to keep everything buttoned up or controlled.
* Overdone vintage clothing and shoes may simply make you look out-of-date.

* Thinly strapped mules may make you look as if you're not on solid footing.
* Skimpy, thinly strapped sandals may make you look like you let it all hang out.
* Scuffed or worn shoes definitely make you look sloppy.

casual blunders

Just say "no" to casual Fridays

My best advice: When in doubt, don't wear it. If you're standing in front of your bedroom mirror asking yourself if you look like you're heading to a sporting event instead of work, then definitely do not wear this outfit to the place where you earn your daily bread. Particularly in corporate environments, failing to look smartly pulled together can send negative messages: you have problems making decisions; you're ineffective at project coordination; or you lack of presentation skills.

 is that a shoe in your pocket . . . .

In 1468, the Pope declared *poulaines* (cloth shoes with toes so long and tapering that owners had to stuff the toes with horsehair to retain their shape) lewd and vain. Despite his objections, these phallic symbols remained wildly popular with the courtiers and lasted until their novelty wore out and commoners adopted them. These shoes reincarnated centuries later in Britain in the form of spike-toed shoes called "winkle-pickers." Juvenile British rockers in the 1950s also considered "winkle-pickers" highly sexually suggestive.

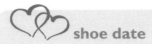 **shoe date**

Time to break out of a corporate state of mind and party! Call your girlfriends and invite them to bring clothes, shoes, and accessories to swap. Beforehand, write some clever story requirements on individual slips of paper and stuff them into a pair of pumps. For example: Where did you buy your first pair of shoes? What shoes were you wearing when you surrendered your virginity? Where did you make your most recent shoe purchase, and how much did you pay? Where did your best friend buy those sexy pumps, and how much did she pay for them? Where can you find affordable Blahnik knockoffs? Who has the best sales? When does Macy's put designer shoes on sale? After settling in, start the fun by having each friend withdraw a story requirement. When she shares her hard-won shoe wisdom, she can exchange something she brought for someone else's treasure.

Work studies have shown that casually dressed employees send the wrong message to clients. When clients see sloppily dressed employees, they tend to equate this with a lack of professionalism and wonder if the firm has the level of professionalism they desire. They may even wonder if they can trust the firm with their projects.

Even if your company has adopted a "casual Friday" policy, dressing way down is simply not a good idea if you're in a corporate environment, such as a law firm, banking institution, and real estate or consulting firms—no matter what everyone else does. Like it or not, particularly in urban areas, as soon as recent economic strictures led to increased competition for jobs, dressing up surged in popularity. It is simply too easy for your boss to interpret an increasingly casual presentation as a slackening attitude about professionalism.

You can dress down, but do it with immense style and only to a certain point, stopping far short of jeans and ordinary sneakers.

The logical exception, of course, is if you work in a factory, a workshop, a health club, or an industry that ordinarily requires jeans, sneakers, and T-shirts. If you work in a creative industry—fashion, art, publishing, advertising, etc.—clean, expensive, stylish jeans worn with high-quality boots or shoes, including vintage leather sneakers or stylish, athletically styled lace-ups, and an expensive, classy blouse, a silk T-shirt, or a sweater set may pass muster, but you're still better off to limit them to the *occasional* casual Friday. If you adore your vintage sneakers, shake it up and wear them with expensive, tailored trousers, creating a hip rather than a casual image.

Sabrina Lyle, who worked in a casual business environment in Alabama, discovered the underlying power in wearing fabulous footwear. "Twenty-five years ago, I bought a pair of Dexter cowboy boots for about $90, and although I rarely wear them and had virtually forgotten how much I loved them, I still own them. I had also forgotten how much I loved boots until a few years ago when I stopped by a biannual kids' clothing swap sale with a coworker and spied what looked to be a single pair of women's boots peeking out of a pile of kids' shoes on a trestle table. I wasn't looking for anything, but they caught my eye. I walked over and pulled out a pair of leather/suede, 3-inch stacked heel, stitched and etched, steel-toed white Zodiac cowboy boots wrapped in a large Ziploc bag. Although they must have cost $200 new, a piece of masking tape listed their price as $3.00, and they were in my size!

"I got so excited; I literally jumped up and down, startling the coworker who had taken me to the sale. She had no idea what those boots meant to me. It felt like karma to find those boots; like some incredibly lucky break. In fact, those spunky boots quickly came to represent liberation and renewal. This coworker had a tendency to dominate me, and, although silent up to that point, I was already buckling myself in for a fight. When I wore the boots a few days later, teamed with blue jeans and a blazer, she drew back and took a second look. My high-heeled, white cowboy boots gave me a feeling of power; I walked taller and straighter; I felt stronger, clearer, more myself in full power and glory. Whatever insecurities held me back almost magically diminished.

"I don't know if it was the boots, per se, but within months of buying those Zodiac boots and walking taller, I gathered enough confidence to quit that job—where my dominating coworker and others were always telling me what to do, second-guessing me, and watching my every move—and return to school to pursue my real dreams. Whatever happened when I wore those boots helped me remember that I could stand on my own two feet and somehow gave me the gumption to do so. I've worn those boots so often in the last two years everyone who knows me identifies them with me, and every one of them has heard the story of my karma boots."

If casual is perfectly acceptable at your place of business, it's still wise to follow these guidelines:

* Casual never means sloppy, hasty, indifferent, lazy, indiscriminate, or unkempt.
* If you do wear jeans, avoid anything ripped, frayed, studded, or dirty.

* No stretched, faded, ripped, or decorated T-shirts (no logos, no ornate rhinestones).
* No scuffed, worn, or dirty shoes . . . ever!
* No common sneakers; high-fashion, immaculate sneakers are okay in rare situations.
* No clunky clogs or slippery mules.
* No thongs and no flip-flops . . . ever!

the stiletto rules

When to wear them to the office—and when not to

If we define a stiletto as any thinly shaped heel that exceeds 3 inches in height, the first thing you want to consider is whether they send a message of, or actually create, imbalance. Very few women can walk more than one block, much less thirty times around the office, in stilettos. Unless you're one of them, you may want to wear your stilettos only in date situations when walking can be restricted to bare necessities. They also may be more appropriate for formal business wear, such as an awards dinner or Christmas party.

Whether you consider the assumptions fair or not, in terms of general office wear, keep the following in mind:

* Wearing extremely high heels can send an underlying (unconscious) message that everything you do contains an element of sexual negotiation. Some may also assume you'll go to any heights, even at the risk of dangerously teetering on a precipice. If you want to pack the wallop of heels *and* send a message of

strength, wear 3-inch-heeled closed pumps. Closed pumps give the impression of containment, plus they offer more support than slingbacks, open toes, or sandals.

* Stiletto boots, particularly knee-high or higher, invariably elicit (unconscious) bondage fantasies. If you want to impress your boss with your bravado, opt for more conservatively heeled boots designed to elicit positive warrior images.

* Wearing stilettos while attending or conducting a meeting in a conservative corporate environment can distract from, or even weaken, your professional image. You'll have all the men thinking sexual thoughts and all the women envious. Better to wear red suede, high-heeled pumps with panache.

* Wearing spiky heels and spiky toes may elicit images of you stabbing someone in the back. Save the steely, needle-thin heels and pointy toes for social occasions.

Of course, to every rule, there are exceptions:

* If you work for a company involved in couture, ready-to-wear, advertising, or creative arts businesses, your contemporaries may consider wearing very fashionable stilettos *de rigueur*.

 watch your cleavage

In 1984, even the normally staid *Wall Street Journal* used sexually suggestive language to describe a shoe—*low-cut throat line, which means it shows cracks between the toes or what the industry calls toe cleavage.*

* If you work in an industry where being female is a plus, stilettos, as long as they aren't blatantly sexual or flamboyant, will increase your power quotient.
* If you are in a situation where maximizing your femininity works in your favor, wearing stilettos will set you apart from the pack. Still, to avoid negative assumptions, opt for moderately thin heels and fairly conservative uppers.

a strutting business plan
Enhance your professional image without breaking the bank

The first step in creating a Strutting Business Plan involves identifying your corporate culture and its specific wardrobe requirements. Basically, today's business world has broad classifications, as follows.

Classic Business Attire
You wear mix-and-match suits; dresses worn with suit jackets; conservative, low to mid-heel pumps; and conservative, top-quality boots and slip-ons with pants, always with hosiery. If you are in a particularly creative field or fashion, you may incorporate a few, carefully selected high-fashion items.

Best shoes: Low-cut, plain pumps in smooth leather with matching heel and sole on slender, medium-height heels.
Office don'ts: No boots with classic suits. No patents, no metallic leathers, no sporty styles. Slingbacks only in summer or when they match the outfit (such as two-tone or matching piping).

Contemporary-Classic Business Attire

This type of workplace allows for loosening of the suit rule, though jackets are preferable on meeting days. More casual pants suits are acceptable, as are sweaters and blouses worn with pants and skirts; simple, yet professional dresses; well-groomed pumps, slingbacks, ballet flats, loafers, and dressy sandals in the summer, usually worn with stockings.

Best shoes: Classic pumps, loafers, oxfords, and boots. Slingbacks and open toes acceptable, particularly in warm weather. Fabric shoes when they match the outfit.

Office don'ts: No denim, no athletic; may include some fashion items, such as a leather jacket.

Informal Business Attire

You wear high-quality pants and skirts, blouses/sweaters, summer dresses, and sleeveless tops. Wearing jackets and stockings wins brownie points.

Best shoes: Well-groomed shoes, loafers, flats, sandals; no stockings okay in summer (as long as feet are immaculate).

Office don'ts: Denim (wear it only if it *truly* is okay with the boss); no athletic gear.

Artistic/Creative Business Attire

Lucky you! Eclectic and personality rule the day. There is a loosening of all strictures, with requisite individualism in your workplace. A need to win fashion acclaim pressures you to create favorable, distinctive, memorable impressions.

Best shoes: Anything goes! Trendsetting clothing and footwear assembled in unconventional ways, unique combinations, mixture of textures, fabrics, moods. Decorated denim and athletic, vintage with a twist, and bold coloring all play a role.

Fashion don'ts: Boring sneakers and shoes, out-of-date shoes (if you're in this category, you know the difference between *trés* cool vintage and outdated!), raggedy or scuffed shoes.

Once you have identified your category, refer back to your wardrobe assessment in Chapter 3, noting what your specific needs are in relation to creating an ideal corporate footwear wardrobe.

In Chapter 8, we'll delve even deeper into your closet to assess real versus imagined needs and help you create a plan for buying the shoes you'll need to meet your corporate needs. The best plan involves starting out slow and building upon what you already have. Again, buy the best quality you can afford and keep reaching higher in terms of your wardrobe and your professional goals.

changing times

In July 1939, *Vogue* magazine referred to open sandals as "skeletonized shoes." They opined that open toes and open heels were not for city wear and said sandals were only appropriate after 5 P.M. with cocktail dresses or summer evening wear.

When matching shoes with clothing, consider the following guidelines:

* Straight-leg pants look best with high heels or thinly soled boots.
* Wide-legged pants look best with low to medium-height, stacked-heel ankle boots, lace-up oxfords, or sturdy loafers.
* Cropped pants look best with ballet flats or loafers.
* Miniskirts look best with low-heeled shoes or knee-high boots.
* Full skirts look best with substantial, yet tapered heels.
* A-line skirts look best with medium-heeled pumps or knee-high boots.
* Pencil skirts look best with medium to high-heeled pumps or slingbacks.
* Long skirts look best with wedges, stacked heels, or thickly-heeled boots.

shoe savvy

What shoes to wear to work

We've agreed at this point that classic pumps (1- to 3-inch heels, closed vamp) are the ultimate professional business accessory, but stylish oxfords, loafers, boots, and slingbacks also are very appropriate in most situations. Again, steering away from sexually charged shoes or overly casual shoes provides a more professional image. Otherwise, exercising style variation is an excellent idea and encouraged in all corporate environments. Guidelines for refining your Business Strutting Plan include the following.

✳ Wearing all black can be overpowering. If your suit is black, consider shoes that highlight an accent color (red silk blouse with red suede pumps; electric blue silk tank with black pumps piped in electric blue; green silk scarf with green suede boots).

✳ Cleverly matching shoes and boots to your outfit makes you look polished.

✳ Shoes and boots need to make the same fashion statement as your outfit. Unless done very cleverly, trendy paired with classic may leave people questioning your taste discernment.

✳ Wear sneakers to walk to the office, but always change into your office shoes as soon as you arrive. (Men—*bosses*—tend to discount women wearing athletic shoes in the workplace.)

✳ Knee-high, patent leather boots may be too sexy for the office. In general, limit patent leathers to ankle boots, loafers, oxfords, and sandals, or as an additional tone on plain leather or suede pumps and boots.

✳ Lightweight skirts and dresses require lightweight shoes; heavy clothing requires stockier shoes or boots for proper balance.

✳ Only wear chunky shoes when they are essential to your total look; when paired with a heavy knit sweater, tweed skirt, and sweater tights, for example.

✳ Limit loafers and oxfords to pants. In general, they do not work with knee to mid-calf skirts, long skirts, or skirts with a slit.

✳ Embellished shoes are most appropriate when they are an expression of your creativity and indigenous to your field—fashion, art, advertising, etc.

* Pair turtlenecks and long pants with loafers, oxfords, or boots (never with sandals).
* Slingbacks, sandals, open toes, or shoes with cutouts look their best when paired with nude hosiery or bare legs.

So, girls, as you're learning, shoes definitely make the woman. Now that we've shod you for maximum impact at work, it's time to take our play just as seriously as we do the climb up that corporate ladder. As we move into the next chapter, it's time to don your workout clothes and meet me at the gym!

7

the skinny on athletic shoes

> There is a spiritual virtue and value that are implied
> by athletic shoes. You can't slink like you can in a
> stiletto, so it represents a new form of femininity. It
> implies a new kind of strength.
>
> Anne Hollander, author of <u>Seeing Through Clothes</u>

now that we've covered your bedroom and the boardroom, it's time to discuss your leisure time. When it comes to athletic/casual footwear, we'll focus on ways to spruce up your wardrobe, express your personality, and feminize your ultra-casuals. *Change Your Shoes, Change Your Life* means adopting and projecting *shoe attitude* in all realms. Why settle for boring sneakers, when you can find fantastic athletic shoes that allow you to walk, run, and jump farther and faster while looking fabulous? The more you solidify your *shoe attitude* and thereby revitalize your life, the more you'll want to *strut your stuff* in style. So, move it, shake it, jiggle it, and race it. Exercise is not only empowering and energizing, it reconnects mind, body, and soul, freeing you to express your ultimate femininity. So, let's talk fashionable, functional sneakers to maximize your sex appeal while you maximize your physical assets.

the genesis of sneakers

During the early days of the twentieth century, fashion generated from couturier designers, primarily Parisian couturier designers, and trickled down to mainstream America. One of the first companies to shake that tree originated in California in the late 1800s when Levi Strauss, in concert with Jacob Davis, created riveted denim pants and almost single-handedly revolutionized American fashion. Adopted by cowboys working the range and gold miners flocking to California, jeans became synonymous with rugged men who wore them for utilitarian purposes. During World War II, women donned denim overalls to join the labor force, but the real boom in denim came in the 1960s when counterculture hippies claimed them as their dominant anti-establishment uniform. While haute couture snubbed jeans—they are still an anomaly in Paris—Americans adored jeans and incorporated them into their everyday lives, setting the pace for the rest of the world. In recent years, Paris haute couture reluctantly embraced jeans, evidenced by a $3,000 pair created by longtime Gucci designer Tom Ford.

Like Levi's, sneakers began their upward trajectory toward Paris *haute couture* on the streets of America. Hollywood not only introduced glamour; it also introduced sportswear to the world. Images of healthy Californians, including Katherine Hepburn and Cary Grant, leading idyllic lives in casual clothing made their way around the world, instantly popularizing tennis shoes and sportswear. For better or worse, the casual lifestyle, and its accompanying wardrobe, became a worldwide phenomenon.

Although sneakers were adopted by counterculture groups, epitomized by James Dean in his Jack Purcells, the majority of men and women continued to wear sneakers only when participating in sporting activities. However, as our culture loosened its dress strictures in the 1970s, casual clothing and shoes gained in prominence. When the city's transit workers went on strike in 1980, thousands of New York City women donned sneakers for their long walks to work and created a revolution. About the same time, aerobics took the country by storm, inspiring Reebok to create the Freestyle, the first athletic sneaker specifically designed for women. Comfort-stretch clothing and colored aerobic shoes were simply irresistible and quickly led to a popular explosion of casual wear.

 sneaker fads

Rebel with a cause James Dean lived in his Jack Purcells.
The ever-creative Woody Allen favored red Converse high-tops.
Artist Andy Warhol ran around Manhattan in tattered Keds.
Starsky & Hutch popularized Adidas Dragons.
Fast Times at Ridgemont High popularized Vans.
Back to the Future II popularized Nike Custom.

By this point, trends bubbled up from the streets; musicians, urban teens, and the counterculture effectively broke the couture spell. At least as often as they arose from Paris, fashion trends now emerged from popular culture: music, movies, celebrities, and grassroots movements in the streets. Splinter groups, such as soccer fans in Europe, skateboarders in America, indie rockers, and hip-hop and rap artists generated their own styles, styles which rapidly progressed up through the ranks to mainstream culture. Sneakers—particularly vintage sneakers—developed mass cachet, becoming so popular that the term *sneaker pimp* gained favor as a way to describe someone so obsessed with sneakers they collect them. Even more so than other footwear, sneaker fads fly hot and fast, becoming ubiquitous as soon as people outside the tribe start wearing them *en masse*. Athletic sneakers eventually became such potent status symbols, people judged others by the quality and

 deadstock

Deadstock refers to vintage, never-worn sneakers still in their original boxes. The popularity of vintage sneakers has generated an industry, with many styles gaining the status of collectibles widely traded on the Internet. Some hot brands include Adidas joggers, Roms, Mercury Players, Chuck T's, Air Jordans, Furys, Rifts, Omega Flamers, Blazers, Bruins, Puma Clydes, Run DMC high-tops, Puma Jams, Vans (Checkerboards, Off the Wall, and Crackled). Visit these Web sites:

vintageusa.com   *snapsorama.com*
ebay.com   *sneakerking.com*
deadshoescrolls.com   *sneakerpimp.com*

swoosh me

In 1971, Phil Knight, cofounder of Nike, commissioned a graphic design student to develop a logo for Nike's new line of trainers. He wanted a symbol of movement, which inspired Carolyn Davidson to create what became the famous Nike swoosh. Knight wasn't thrilled with her design but succumbed to a pressing deadline, commenting at the time "It will grow on me." He paid Davidson $35 at the time, but in 1983, after the extraordinary success of the line and its inspirational swoosh, Knight awarded Davidson a diamond-encrusted swoosh ring and handed her an envelope containing sizable Nike stock.

fashion of their sneakers. As such, hard-to-get foreign and vintage American styles became the essence of cool.

In 1992, the corporate offices of Alcoa, an aluminum manufacturing company in Pittsburgh, officially sanctioned casual Fridays, opening the door for employees to dress down in offices all across the country. In 1995, IBM adopted a casual work week, reflecting America's increasingly informal manner of dressing. Thus began the days of fanny packs, T-shirts, jeans, khakis, and sneakers. As the casual bandwagon rolled merrily along, stores like The Gap, Banana Republic, and Old Navy played both ends of the economic spectrum by creating a hip, modern image, epitomized by Sharon Stone pairing a Gap T-shirt with a fancy ball-gown skirt at the 1995 Oscars.

Endorsements by athletes also contributed to the mass popularity of certain sneakers. Early on, Chuck Taylor immortalized Converse All-Stars; in the 1980s, Michael Jordan immortalized Nike's Air Jordans. The first women to win endorsement contracts

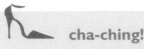

cha-ching!

Although male athletes unfairly earn astronomically more than female athletes, Venus and Serena Williams have finally moved into the upper echelon of endorsement deals. Serena currently pulls in $6 million a year, while sister Venus landed a five-year contract that pulls in $8 million a year—that's a whopping $40 million! You go, girls!

were Chris Evert for Converse and Virginia Wade for PRO-Keds. By the early 1990s, athletic endorsements were so successful that Nike began changing its styles every six months to create fashion demand.

Female endorsements, however, continued to lag far behind. During the 1996 Olympics, when the American women's soccer team won the gold, the tide turned. Suddenly all eyes turned to female athletes, and stars like Mia Hamm, Jackie Joyner-Kersee, Nancy Kerrigan, and Monica Seles won lucrative contracts. Around the same time, the popularity of the Women's Basketball Association (WNBA) inspired Nike to create the first female signature shoe, the Air Swoops, in honor of Sheryl Swoops. Because

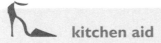

kitchen aid

When running gained popularity in the early 1970s, Bill Bowerman, a running coach, wanted a lighter shoe. As an experiment, he placed a piece of rubber into a waffle iron, which was so successful in lightening the rubber, he took the idea to Phil Knight at Nike. Together, they revolutionized the running-shoe market.

women were spending $5.4 billion, or $200 million more than men, on athletic shoes, it was a wise move. By the late 1990s, Nike had 50 female athletes contracted for endorsements!

yes, virginia, there are specific shoes for specific sports

Sports fans identify personally with the athletes; you put yourself in the players' sneakers, experiencing their trials and triumphs as your own . . . But when you're a chick, sometimes it's hard to put yourself in someone else's sneakers . . . Now that women are playing professionally, it's a whole other ball game. Apathetic, pathetically femmey gals like me are now able to "get it"—to experience the thrill of sports, to admire the strategy, speed, and skill involved. For the first time in our lives, we're seeing ourselves on the playing field—as national heroes.

Susan Jane Gilman, author of <u>Kiss My Tiara</u>

Different sport activities require different sport shoes—walking, running, tennis, dance, basketball, baseball, soccer, golf, skiing, and on and on. In many cases, your shoes will be the most important piece of sports equipment you purchase. A wise choice will prevent pain and injury, not only to your feet, but to the rest of your body. The four most important elements to consider are the amount of support needed, the level of comfort, durability of the footwear, and how much the shoe assists foot movements needed to perform the sport.

There are as many types of athletic shoes as there are sports, and it is preferable that you buy the appropriate shoes for each sport. Athletic-shoe designers work for years to create shoes that maximize comfort, support, flexibility, and protection. Take advantage of their knowledge, girls! It also is wise to research your options prior to purchase, seek assistance from knowledgeable sales staff, and adhere to the golden rule of shoe shopping: buy the best quality shoes you can reasonably afford. Top-quality athletic shoes will cost significantly more than $50, but they'll last you the equivalent of 500 miles. Removable inserts, which you can replace several times a year, can help extend the lifespan of the shoes. When trying on athletic shoes, always try on both shoes and lace them. Stand, walk, squat, and even run around the store a few times before making your decision.

You need court shoes for any sport that requires quickness, side-to-side or lateral movements, and some bouncing. Court shoes include tennis shoes, basketball shoes, squash shoes, racquetball shoes, and volleyball shoes. They will adequately protect your feet by providing increased stability and flexibility.

Running puts three times as much stress on your feet as does ordinary walking, so it's super-important to buy the right sneakers for this sport. Conscientious running shoe designers create shoes that will redistribute your weight for maximum shock absorption and provide additional cushioning and stability. Leather and suede provide increased durability and allow your feet to breathe. If you are a runner, replace your running shoes after 300 to 500 miles—or every six months—to maintain maximum shock absorption. You change the oil in your car every three months; why not apply the same loving maintenance to your feet?

sssh

Vintage, foreign, and hard-to-find sneakers are so hot that the Alfie Rivington Club in New York City has garnered an exclusive clientele. It's one of the few resources where you can find sneakers that aren't available anywhere else in the world. Unfortunately, they have neither a storefront nor a sign. You have to know someone who knows where to find their doorbell.

Other sports that require sport-specific footwear include ballet, aerobics, racewalking, regular walking, soccer, golf, and skiing. But the best thing about all these specialized shoes is that you can wear them just for fun. You don't have to be a runner to wear a phat pair of trainers.

who said you had to run in them?

I have several pairs of sneakers, none of which I really need. I don't run or play tennis or even belong to a gym. In fact, all of my sneakers were chosen for their looks, the same way I choose all my other shoes.

Nancy MacDonell Smith, author of <u>The Classic Ten</u>

Like jeans, sneakers traveled far beyond their original purpose and far beyond the streets where they began. Expensive sneakers implied that you had plenty of time and money to pursue sporting activities. They went from casual shoes to status symbols, objects of obsession, and even cause for aggression. In 1990, Nike's Air Jordans soared over $100 at retail, leading, in urban areas, to instances of theft, both from shoe stores and, in a few cases, directly from the owners' feet!

What all that means is that a wide variety of sneakers have become hot fashion items. Most of them are deadly comfortable and there's a proliferation of styles to choose from, so there's no reason why you can't replace boring sneakers with fashionable ones or their upscale cousins—running shoes, tennis shoes, or bowling shoes—for all your casual needs. In fact, you'll look far more with it if you've made the leap from utilitarian sneakers to hot sneakers for day-to-day wear. The hotter the sneaker, the more you can justify wearing it in a multitude of settings. A fabulous pair of vintage red Pumas, for example, can look great with jeans for any casual occasion, but you can also wear them with a snazzy pair of black slacks for art gallery openings, grocery shopping, Saturday brunch with your girlfriends, or running errands in the city. If the sneakers are snappy enough, and you've pulled together an outfit that coordinates or attractively offsets them, you'll always look *au courant*.

My niece, Michele Kaczmarek, a laboratory science specialist living and working in Washington, D.C., adores athletic shoes. "Because I have size 11 feet, the only time I had fun shopping for shoes came when I found a specialized athletic shoe store that actually had an incredible array of sizes in stock. The salesperson spent at least a half hour with me, and even convinced me to inch up in size for maximum fit! Surprisingly, they had a large selection in size 12s, which meant—for one of the first times in my life—I actually had the chance to try on a number of shoes and choose something truly appealing. They may not have been the sexiest shoes in the world, but for once I felt like I had finally bought a pair of shoes that were truly mine . . . I loved them!

"Even though I attended rival North Carolina State, and these running shoes were Carolina blue, as soon as I slipped them on, I felt like I was walking on air. I can run for miles without feeling tired or worrying about shin splints. They also have a mesh upper I find extremely comfortable that also allows my feet to breathe. They are so fabulous they make me feel sexy, or at least as if a bit of footwear pizzazz is finally available to me."

just do it—you can run in them!

We all know the benefits of girls playing sports. We know that it fosters confidence and coordination, teamwork skills and physical strength. Studies have shown that young women who play are more likely to do better in math and science, and less likely to become sexually active at a young age or stay with a guy who beats them.

Susan Jane Gilman, author of Kiss My Tiara

In the 1970s, women made tremendous strides in the career marketplace and in the sporting arenas. We ran our homes, our families, our careers, and our lives, balancing these roles, gaining ground, *and* exercising—all with aplomb. And why wouldn't we? Exercising not only benefits your health, it bolsters your sense of self-possession and confidence, qualities that make a woman even more attractive. An athletic woman is a sexy woman, a woman who loves her body and knows how to move. Muscular bodies are graceful bodies, and what's sexier than grace?

From the 1970s on, female athletic participation in the realm of professional sports increased at unprecedented levels. When Nike launched the slogan "Just Do It" in 1988, more and more liberated

nike comeback

Even when you think athletic shoes are so over, they have a way of filtering back in. Nike's Air Max had fallen out of favor in the mid 1990s, so the fashionistas adopted Nike's new color-graduated 1995 Air Max sneakers as their "anti-label." By the time Nike introduced its silver mesh version in January 1997, the sneakers had become so *haute couture*, the shoes shot up in price to four digits. Gwen Stefani and Madonna helped catapult them into mainstream, and they became so scarce, a style reporter for the *New York Times* wrote a column about his four-month search for a pair.

and empowered American women were embracing endurance sports. Because female athletes were rightfully taking their place alongside the best male athletes in the world, Nike's slogan was the perfect battle cry for professional and casual sports enthusiasts.

Today, we have a long list of female role models in sports, and they inspire us to greater heights. Serena Williams, for example, possesses a bold sense of style, so much so she rattled the fairly conservative tennis world when she marched onto court wearing a black denim miniskirt and knee-high, black patent boots over her court shoes. The boots enhanced Serena's already exceptional physical prowess and skill, which both unnerved her opponent and declared to the world that Serena was ready for battle. As she slowly unbuckled those boots, commentators noted the psychological impact—equating her to a supremely confident warrior marching into battle. Serena, who wore jazzy court shoes for the actual tournament, later found the hullabaloo over her fashionable boots amusing, and cast all discussion aside by explaining that she simply wore the boots because she loved them.

So make like Serena and wear your favorite sports shoes—run in them, walk in them, play tennis in them, play soccer or golf or squash—and look like one of the coolest girls on the planet while you're doing it. Shine everywhere; it's your right.

hello, comfortable does not mean ugly!

The sneaker has become part of the library of necessary items for most women's wardrobes.

Daryl Kerrigan, Harper's Bazaar

The good news is that sneakers are extremely comfortable, and therefore good for your feet, and today the wealth of styles available makes it easy to find groovy ones for all your needs. The use of color, fabrications like suede or shiny patents, stripes, logos, straps, and even rhinestones has revolutionized the sports shoe market. If you're not making a fashion statement in your choice of sneakers, you're not working hard enough!

Warren Thayer, editorial director for a trade publication and once-upon-a-time a fellow *Footwear News* editor, actually prefers women in sensible shoes. "If a sexy woman is wearing extremely high heels, I definitely find myself staring at her, intrigued, but at the same time feeling oddly repelled. It's more than twenty years since I was actively dating, but, before I married, I chased my share of high-heeled, come-hither women only to discover that oftentimes they were loosely moral, self-centered, and high-maintenance. When it came time to choose a life partner, I was attracted to women in comfortable, casual shoes, and definitely found women in sneakers quite appealing. They didn't tend to live a pretentious life; they were who they were, and, frankly, they were often better in bed. Or at the very least, I found it easier to have a real conversation with them in the morning."

So, girls, get out there and jog around in your sexy sneakers. You won't have trouble finding absolutely adorable choices. In recent years, high-fashion designers jumped on the sneaker/trainer bandwagon. Jil Sander, Stella McCartney, Prada, Yohji Yamamoto, Paul Smith, Neil Barrett, Donna Karan, Dolce & Gabbana, and even Chanel have either designed shoes for the major athletic brands, such as Adidas, Puma, and Reebok, or added athletic-inspired designs to their repertoire. Sneakers have made the ultimate journey from legitimate sports to the street, to fashion, to *haute couture*. Designers, models, actresses, high-profile businesswomen, and journalists have all de-formalized their casual wear and joined the world in its love of sneaker comfort for casual wear. When Hermès created The Quick in 1998, it quickly sold out in Paris and New York at $525 a pair. Gucci, Prada, and Chanel hustled to catch up. Stella McCartney, who loves to mix it up, wears her athletic shoes with flowered dresses and diamond bangles!

 the rich do it

In 2004, Reebok opened a Beverly Hills retail store to offer expensive versions of their most popular styles. On opening day, they featured a $1,000 pair of hot-pink crocodile sneakers. "The rich and famous love our brand," a spokesperson explained.

happy feet are powerful feet
A guide for girl jocks

When it comes to athletics, choosing the appropriate, specially designed shoes for your particular sport, buying the right size, and protecting and pampering your feet will go a long way toward preventing injuries. Since body-weight and impact pressure greatly increases during any sporting activity, wearing shoes designed specifically for the sport will greatly increase protection. For basic information on selecting properly fitting shoes, please review *Making Sure the Shoe Fits* in the Appendix. When it comes to athletic shoes, however, it would be wise to pay attention to these additional suggestions:

* Select soft, pliable materials that provide maximum flexibility.
* Make sure your athletic shoes bend where your toes bend. Shoes that bend in the middle of the foot increase heel pressure, leaving your Achilles tendon susceptible to injury, especially during high-pressure activities such as running and jumping.
* Adjust fit and comfort cushioning as needed. Prefabricated gel-cushioned pads increase shock absorption, thereby reducing injured tendons and stress fractures.

If you are experiencing pain or discomfort related to your sporting activities or athletic footwear, that's not good! Please reference the fabulously informative orthopedic resources listed in the Appendix for further, very specific information about injuries and proper treatment of injuries. Remember, you should always address foot problems with your physician the minute they arise!

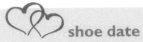

shoe date

Shoe-shopping time! Often we don't give enough consideration to how we dress during our leisure time. Call your Fairy Godmother, and plan a shopping excursion to fabulous athletic clothing and footwear departments. Choose several trendy outfits and then select the most colorful, fun athletic shoes you can find to try on with them. If you find something you love, buy it! Who knows—doing so may inspire you to beef up physical activities in your life, and that's a good, good thing. You go, girls!

the care and feeding of athletic feet

If you are a sporting enthusiast, you'll want to protect your feet from injury by heeding the following.

Learn to Love Warm-Up Stretches

Prior to a workout, to keep your feet flexible and minimize risk of injury, warm up through a series of gentle stretches designed to elongate the foot, ankle, and leg muscles. Post-exercise, repeat the same stretches to cool down.

Elongate Your Ligament

The plantar fascia, an extension of the Achilles tendon, is a tough ligament-like sheet of tissue—extending from the heel bone to the base of the toes—that you can easily injure, resulting in pain and inflammation. To minimize risk of injury, stand on a bottom step with your heels hanging off the edge. Slowly lower your heels until your calf muscles noticeably elongate. Hold the stretch a minimum of ten seconds, working your way slowly, over time, to holding it sixty seconds. Repeat this stretch four times a day, every day.

Boost Circulation

If you want to keep your tootsies in the pink, pump up circulation through regular physical activity. If you can't run, walk, girls,

 shoe do

It's time for a foot spa! Begin with luscious warm-water soaking. Epsom salts will detoxify, reduce swelling, and alleviate pain, but herbal remedies are simply divine and can be equally soothing. Suggested ingredients to create your own combinations:

- *Cleansing/Disinfectants*
  apple cider vinegar, aloe vera oil, calendula oil, lemon juice, chamomile, grapefruit seed oil, witch hazel
- *Anti-inflammatory/Comforting*
  camphor oil, Epsom salts (detoxifies), eucalyptus oil (cools and soothes), ginger (rejuvenates), green tea (decreases swelling), horse chestnut, peppermint oil
- *Itching*
  primrose oil, olive oil (hardens cuticles, softens skin); aloe vera oil

After soaking, dry each foot thoroughly, apply your favorite lotion, and pull on a pair of thin cotton socks. Foot massagers, particularly ones with little rolling balls, are heavenly. Afterward, lie down with your feet elevated for fifteen minutes. If your tootsies still ache, apply arnica cream, wrap your feet in warm towels, elevate fifteen minutes, and then follow with ice packs. *Hint: Do this regularly!*

walk. Other ways to maximize healthy circulation: don't smoke, keep your feet warm, and don't sit for long periods of time with your legs crossed.

Pamper Your Feet

When exercising, or in situations in which your feet sweat, wear moisture-wicking socks to keep your feet clean and dry. Always cover any open wounds, and regularly soak, massage, and apply moisturizing lotion to your feet.

Now that you know how to boost your *shoe attitude* in the bedroom, the boardroom, and on the playing field, we'll move into the second phase of our makeover. We'll begin by going back to your shoe closet to really dig deep to find out who you've been and start dreaming about who you want to be. We're going *plan your strut so you can strut your plan* and really turn your life upside down. Are you ready, girls?

8

back to the shoe closet

The truth is we need Barbie dolls for grown ups too. All our lives would be enriched by having a fantasy doll we could strip naked and dress in our own dreams.

Erica Jong, novelist

ow that we've covered *shoe attitude* and given concrete ways—in your sex life, at work, and at play—to change your life by changing your shoes, this section will address strategic action when it comes to tackling your entire closet. It's time to really clean house, redefine and refine your desired image, and truly revamp your flagging *shoe attitude*. It's time to return to the closet to revisit your clothing and shoes, see what's working and what's not working, immediately eliminate the duds, and generate a plan to create your dream closet. Toward the end of the chapter, we'll discuss your needs, your budget, and your priorities.

We're going to begin by crawling into the nooks and crannies of your closet to figure out who you've been, who you want to be, and how best to get there. As we sift through its contents, keep in mind that your closet represents a collective view of your life—your experiences, your hopes, your ambitions, your dreams, even your sensuality. As you objectively and dispassionately sift through your wardrobe, ask yourself whether you are in search of a new self or simply in search of new shoes. Are you happy with your real self, or do you long to create your ideal self?

If you're relatively happy with your life and only need refresher shoes, your task is far easier—more a matter of mixing and matching.

 are you a shoe-a-holic?

Look for these telltale signs:

You still own your first pair of black patent Mary Janes.

You had your wedding shoes picked out by age fourteen.

You've moved at least five times and have never thrown a pair of shoes away.

You consider shoe shopping a religious experience.

Your friends cringe when you ask them to go shoe shopping.

You buy plain pumps at regular price.

You own a pair of yellow shoes.

You check out other women's feet/legs/ankles more than your boyfriend/husband does.

You have a closetful of shoes and only three outfits to go with them.

You gave your mother designer shoes for Christmas.

Your friends gave you a pillow with "Imelda Marcos Wannabe" embroidered on it.

However, if you are determined to alter your sense of self, you'll need to dig deeper, figure out who you are now, who you want to be, and how you can best achieve the transformation. In both cases, you need to go back to your closet to determine your primary areas for expansion, reorganization, and creativity. Let's begin by discussing your overall fashion personality.

fashion personality

While the archetypal, *Strutting Hall of Fame* images outlined in Chapter 4 are all worth emulating, particularly to express various aspects of your life, your basic fashion personality probably falls into one of the following, more general categories:

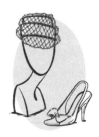

Classic
You want to make a good impression, and know how to construct the proper attire to meet every situation. You consider accessories an indulgence and don't believe in extraordinary measures to achieve a polished elegance (no fireworks for you!). You think long term, shop with a plan, only buy the best, and self-monitor.

A really well-dressed woman in her afternoon clothes should be able to pass through a motley crowd unnoticed, but should create a mild sensation on entering a drawing room among the knowing elite.

Coco Chanel

Contemporary Classic

You're an extroverted classic, keenly aware of the latest fashion currents, and you like to incorporate them—elegantly—into your wardrobe. You still believe that less is more, but throw in a dose of up-to-the-minute sophistication, and make a major commitment to style. You enjoy gaining discreet attention when you walk into a room, and you believe in designer labels, coordinating accessories, and finishing touches.

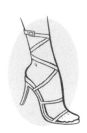

Au Courant

You read all the fashion and celebrity-tracking magazines, know what Jennifer Lopez, Beyoncé, Madonna, and Nicole Kidman are wearing, and always strive to be *au courant*. You prefer buying clothes to buying groceries, and shop until your credit cards are maxed. You familiarize yourself with designer labels and covet many, like making dramatic entrances, and live to win compliments.

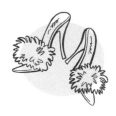

Girly Girl

You dress to reflect your most feminine self, love a girly, feminine approach, and like to spin a web of intrigue. You spend a significant amount of time daydreaming about the man in your life, and are elegantly sexy in public, risqué in private. A goddess by day and femme fatale (or bombshell) by night, you love shoes that elongate your legs and show off your calves and toes.

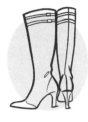

Creative Sparkler

You have many different sides and like to express them all, mixing colors, moods, and textures with free-spirited, yet planned abandon. You have flair, attitude, and pizzazz, express yourself through your wardrobe, celebrate your creativity, and suffer for your art. You are the type of girl who loves exclusivity, and always wear shoes that make a statement.

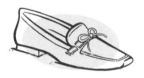

Nature Girl

You care more about your inner self than the outer self you present to the world. You always appear relaxed, unstructured, and completely yourself. You prefer comfort over fashion, possess a low fashion monitor, and need shopping assistance when you have to dress up. At first you may resist, but you need to shake up your world occasionally!

 do you qualify?

Melissa de la Cruz and Karen Robinovitz, authors of a fictional work entitled *The Fashionista Files: Adventures in Four-Inch Heels and Faux Pas,* define a fashionista as "a dedicated follower of fashion ... anyone who has rejected the tried-and-true, staid and sensible, matching-bag-and-shoes, no-white-after-Labor-Day rules to follow a fantasy of art-directed glory." They say fashionistas harbor a deep desire to be "outrageous and over-the-top," explain that she possesses the traits of "a gypsy, a princess, and a diva," and say that she is "a chameleon who will meet every new trend with glee."

Obviously, we are rarely so easily defined, nor should we be; nevertheless, it is helpful to know your basic fashion personality so that you can determine whether your wardrobe works for you or whether it is filled with items that conflict with your basic personality.

clothing

It pains me physically to see a woman victimized, rendered pathetic, by fashion.

Yves Saint Laurent, couturier

All too often, over a long period of time, we accumulate a huge stash of clothing and lose all sight of exactly what we own. If you haven't intentionally reviewed and edited your wardrobe, you probably have dresses you have totally forgotten about, pants you haven't worn for five years, and sweaters, blouses, or jackets so out-of-date you wouldn't dream of wearing them in public. Typically, we have items in our closet that still bear price tags months, and even years, after we purchased them. So why are they still in our closets, taking up valuable space?

Ideally, your clothing, footwear, accessory, and jewelry wardrobe should be a mini-reflection of a designer collection, covering all the bases you need to cover in your life—a few ultra-dressy-event dresses, pantsuits or tuxedos, a significant number of hot date dresses or sexy pantsuits, five to ten appropriate ensembles specific to your career, a sprinkling of slightly-dressed-down business alternatives, three to five casual socializing outfits, five to seven completely casual outfits, and three to five outfits to meet your athletic requirements.

Come, darlings, it's time to creak open your closet door and bring the truths it holds to light. Don't be afraid; you're going to end up in a much better place—one where you love everything that's in your closet, make smart purchases that significantly boost your fashion profile (even while saving you money), and more fully express who you were born to be!

If you own a clothes rack, or two, they are very useful for viewing your clothing throughout the weeding process. To facilitate the process, separate your clothing according to seasonal limitations, function, type of item, and color. For instance, pull all your work dresses out of the closet and hang them on the rack. As you go through them, one by one, ask yourself the following questions:

Is this item serving me now?

If not, do I even like it, or was it a fashion *faux pas*? Remember Cinderella sorting the good lentils from the bad lentils? It's time to be ruthless. If the item isn't working for you, enhancing your life, or cultivating the image you want, please don't hold on to it in hopes that somehow, someday, it will! *Hint*: This also applies to makeup, boyfriends, and jobs.

Does this item reflect and enhance the cohesive image I desire?

As you pull everything out, you'll clearly see where you are now, but is this where you want to be? If not, and the item does not reflect a more adventurous you, chuck it.

Does this item indicate a distinctive style personality?

Of course, you'll want a stable of basics, but you also need items that add punch and ultimately create an enviable fashion personality. If you own ten black skirts, consider eliminating half. Obviously, you want to keep the most fashion-forward, highest-quality items; let the rest go and make a written note not to buy any more black skirts!

Does this item have maximum versatility?

Will it easily mix and match with—and elevate—at least three to five other items in my wardrobe?

If clothing doesn't meet the above criteria, be bold in weeding it out. When you've pared each category down to the keepers, review these clothes carefully, and this time, take notes. By answering the following questions, you can further refine your new image:

* What are your obvious themes—romantic, hard-line career, free-spirited business owner, creative artist, young mother?
* What's missing? Where are the holes? Do you need more date dresses, do you need more classic sheath dresses to wear with your plethora of blazers, do you need sweater sets to freshen up your pencil skirts, do you need updated trousers, or do you need some serious pizzazz?
* What works with what? Does your pink cashmere cardigan bring new life to your favorite black moiré sheath for evening, your navy pin-striped trousers, *and* your chocolate-brown suede

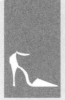

designer dish

David Evins

AMERICAN ICON

David Evins began his career as an illustrator for *Vogue* magazine in the 1930s; they fired him for taking too much artistic license in his drawings. Later, he built a long and successful career designing shoes. He created the jeweled sandals Claudette Colbert wore in *Cleopatra* and the gold brocade mules with turned-up vamps that Elizabeth Taylor wore in a later version of *Cleopatra*. He created a pair of pumps, one shoe red and the other green (signifying maybe yes and maybe no), for Ava Gardner, and also the pumps that Grace Kelly wore when she married Prince Rainier.

pencil skirt for work? Do the five silk blouses you adore need updated trousers and skirts to maximize their appeal? Does the new forest green voile shawl you bought at an art fair successfully dramatize your beige silk trousers, your brown tweed blazer, *and* your strapless black taffeta dress for the opera?

As you work your way through your remaining clothing, a list will emerge that reflects specific items you need in order to create the new you. Pay particular attention to accessories, focusing, of course, on the types of shoes that will add the real spice to your new—or newly reworked—wardrobe. If you own a lot of textured dresses or skirts, you may want to add textured fabrics in shoes and handbags to create a more cohesive style image; if you own a number of monotone sheath dresses, you may want to add bold splashes of color and texture to amplify your fashion quotient.

Continue reviewing your wardrobe information carefully, noticing trends as they develop, and keeping notes (these notes will be invaluable for the fashion *wish book* you'll create in Chapter 9).

 shoe do

Shoes, particularly the types of golden slippers you're going to don, are investments; as such, it's not only prudent to take care of them, but they will only look their best if you expend the small amounts of energy required to maintain them on a regular basis. The rules are pretty simple, and include the following:

- Always use boot shapers or tissue paper or socks to stuff legs of high boots.

- Stuff toes with tissue paper, toe pillows, or socks to maintain shape.

- Always gently brush suede shoes and boots after wearing. Use a pencil eraser to tackle small spots, a bristle brush to loosen dirt, a softer brush to freshen.

- Always remove any dirt or mud from shoes before storing; wipe all leathers and patents with a soft, damp cloth.

- Always polish and buff scuffed shoes before storing.

- Aerate storage boxes to allow leather to breathe.

- Protect shoes and handbags from steam, heat, sunlight, and moisture.

- Apply leather conditioner regularly to maintain suppleness; mink oil is a superb emollient.

- Prior to wearing, rub a polishing cloth repeatedly over toes to shine. (In a pinch, banana peels provide a quick leather shine.)

- Check heels and soles regularly; fix or replace.

- Add rubber soles or taps, as needed for comfort or endurance.

As you compile the information, note what is working for you and what is not working, as well as reasons why it works or doesn't work. For example, if you favor a monochromatic look, your reasons might include an idea that it promotes an easy elegance or that it makes you look taller, trimmer, and polished. It may be working beautifully, or it may not be working because ultimately it makes you forgettable. Your solution may be as simple as adding spectacular shoes and a few scarves, accent pieces, or artistic pieces of jewelry. My friend Jennifer, for example, was so insecure about being petite, she filled her closet with head-to-toe black, brown, and gray ensembles to make her look taller, trimmer, and polished. After being passed over twice for a partnership in her law firm, she wondered if her blacks and browns made her fade into the backdrop at the office. She added spectacular red suede power pumps, several versatile pieces of one-of-a-kind jewelry from a local designer, and a few stunning vintage Pucci scarves. She immediately experienced increased visibility.

It's also important to ask yourself if your clothing is meeting your needs. If you are a young woman in the midst of developing a public relations agency, you may need a wardrobe that reflects a strong business sensibility paired with creative energy and vision. If you are a doctor who has recently begun accepting frequent speaking engagements, you may need a wardrobe that travels well and transmits an authoritarian image. If you are newly single, you may need to sex up your wardrobe to jump-start your own impulses to rejoin the dating scene. Perhaps you have been lackluster in your choices of clothing, shoes, and accessories and you now want to be distinctive; perhaps you endured fashion deprivation and long to finally express the more flamboyant aspects of your personality;

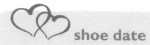

shoe date

Call your Fairy Godmother and entice her to join you for a fantasy shopping excursion. Once you arrive at the high-end boutique or department store of your dreams, each of you embrace the task of selecting three complete—atypical—outfits for the other. Be inventive; choose clothing, shoes, and accessories that are way outside the box for your friend, and ask her to do the same. Take along a digital camera and snap pictures of each other in your fantasy personas. Who knows, you may discover a whole new you!

perhaps you used to think buying inexpensive items stretched your budget but have now realized that buying a few high-quality items will save you more money in the long run.

As a budding singer/songwriter/guitarist who was beginning to perform in local nightclubs, my daughter, Brooke Aved, needed to dramatically spruce up her wardrobe. Because Brooke had always been extremely creative and individualistic, as well as curvaceous, she wanted a feminine, hip look she described as "somewhere between hippie chic and very urban cowgirl." Up to this point, Brooke's closet contained a wide assortment of worn-out jeans, most of which we tossed. She had a tight budget, so we scoured local factory stores. At Ann Taylor, we found fabulous knee-length suede pencil skirts, each with a small ruffle along an uneven hem. Because they were perfect building blocks, and on sale, we bought one in winter white and one in baby blue. We found five sexy, clinging, silk and voile "hippie" tops at Max Studio. For shoes, we found a pair of knee-high, winter white boots and a pair of sexy high-platform sandals, adorned with turquoise beads. We added turquoise hoops, silver dangles, subtly patterned stockings, and an open-weave knit poncho. These simple "basics" solidified a defined image that Brooke could quickly build on. Within weeks, she found a pair of low-cut jeans with a built-in fabric belt, a flared denim miniskirt, a brown suede vest, a pair of brown suede platform sandals, handmade T-shirts, and a cropped denim jacket to expand her professional wardrobe, taking her from bland to sensational.

When I surrendered my public relations job to fly off to Paris to work as a writer and photographer, my own wardrobe also needed major revamping. Because I planned to spend most of my time photographing throughout Paris, I needed sensible pants, comfortable shoes, and layering sweaters. After jettisoning my power clothes and salvaging a few dressy outfits with their coordinating pumps, I bought a minimal wardrobe of stylish, comfortable black trousers. Because I adored The Gap's basic crisp, stretch-cotton blouses and because they fit my need for maximum flexibility and classic good looks, I bought them in four colors. I added a few classic V-neck sweaters, a snazzy denim jacket (with four pockets to hold film canisters), and three pairs of flat shoes: black leather fisherman sandals, brown leather oxfords, and a pair of vintage Nike sneakers. Due to space and budget issues, I purposely limited my wardrobe to absolute essentials and intentionally bought high-quality shoes. Of course, once in Paris, I added a few sexy outfits, but my basic photography wardrobe, and most particularly those expensive, well-made shoes, made it possible for me to comfortably walk all over Paris *and* pass muster with fashion-conscious Parisians.

So, my dears, with these newly gained insights tightly in hand, it's time to talk shoes!

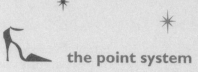 **the point system**

Accumulating Points to Indulge Your Shoe Obsession:

  250 points = one pair of affordable (under $100) fashion shoes

  500 points = one pair of reasonably priced (under $200) shoes

1,000 points = one pair of super-sexy, designer sandals; think stiletto

1,500 points = one pair of just-for-the-hell-of-it shoes
                       (furry mules, snakeskin slides, rhinestone anything, etc.)

2,000 points = one pair of pretty-damn-fabulous boots

2,500 points = one pair of high-heel, designer pumps; think stiletto

3,000 points = one pair of Blahnik, Prada, or Choo pumps or sandals

4,000 points = one pair of thigh-high, designer boots

5,000 points = anything you want, baby

- You immediately got up when your alarm rang: 250 points
- Mother criticizes your clothes: 500 points
- Heel breaks on everyday shoes: 250 points
- Heel breaks on expensive shoes: 500 points
- Your best friend borrowed your sexy sandals: 250 points
- Three women insist on knowing where you bought your shoes: 500 points
- You spy Samantha or Carrie on *Sex and the City* wearing a shoe you already own: 1,000 points
- The man selling you shoes fondles your leg: 500 points
- You spilled red wine on your favorite fabric pumps: 500 points
- You indulged your craving for Godiva twice in one week: 500 points

- You scarf down Twinkies, popcorn, Hershey bars, and a full bottle of cheap red wine while watching sad movies: 1,000 points

- You haven't had sex for three months: 1,000 points

- You had sex recently with a loser: 1,500 points

- You haven't had sex for six months: 2,000 points

- You can't remember the last time you had sex: 3,000 points

- You're fantasizing about Mr. Rogers: 4,000 points

- A man you just met dumps you before you leave the bar: 1,000 points

- A man you dated for six months breaks up with you in person: 2,500 points

- A man you dated for six months breaks up with you over the phone, through a friend, by e-mail, or by leaving a note: 3,500 points

- Men stare at your legs when you pass: 1,000 points

- Men stare at your swaying behind when you pass: 2,000 points

- Your boss whistled when he spotted your latest pumps: 3,000 points

- Your boss fired you for riling up men in the office with your sexy shoes: 4,000 points

- Your fiancé broke off your engagement three months before the wedding: 5,000 points

- Your fiancé broke off your engagement after you spent a small fortune on "lucky" wedding shoes: 10,000 points

shoes

Now that you've gained a strong understanding of your clothing wardrobe, you'll want to review all your post-Chapter-3-purge shoes, analyzing them in the same manner.

* Are these shoes serving me now?
* Do they not only reflect, but truly enhance the cohesive image I desire?
* Do they indicate a desirable, distinctive style personality?
* Do they have maximum versatility?
* Which shoes work particularly well with my wardrobe?
* Where do I need to fill in or experiment?

With shoes, of course, come a new range of questions:

* Do they fit? *If not, they go.*
* Do they flatter your figure, legs, and feet? *If not, they go.*
* Do they enhance your wardrobe? *If not, they go.*
* Do they send the desired message—classy, stylish, vivacious, creative, or ambitious? *If not, they go.*
* Are they cheap? *If yes, they go.* The only exception would be canvas or ultra-casual summer sandals, which are playthings.

Also, more so with shoes than clothes, an emotional element also can play a central role. If you find yourself fondling a pair, turning them over and over in your hot little hands, cringing at any thought of tossing them into the "dispose" pile, you need to take a moment. Think back to when you bought them or when you wore them last. How did you feel when you put them on? Did they represent a certain phase of your life? If so, do they still fit your image or are you clinging to them the same way you might cling to a child-hood teddy bear? Rate the shoes' attraction from 1 to 5, with 1 representing low attraction, and then make your decision. If memories are the prime reason they're still in your closet, get out your digital camera, snap a few snazzy photos, and toss the shoes.

After you have pared down your shoe wardrobe—good girl!—pick up your trusty pad and pencil and review the keepers. Write down your color inventory: You have five pairs of black pumps; you need to add brown, beige, and possibly two pairs of boldly colored pumps; you wear a lot of navy and need alternative neutrals to complement your clothing; you love red, own two red blazers and three red blouses, yet there's not a single pair of red shoes in your closet.

Also record your style findings. You have a closet full of skirts and only two pairs of high-heeled pumps to complement them. You adore color, but every pair of sneakers you own is white with blue or black accents. All of your shoes are smooth leather; you need to add snakeskin, fabric, or suede. You haven't bought a new pair of boots in five years; you need a sharp pair of knee-high black suede boots to spice up your wardrobe.

As you review your clothing and shoes, be sure to notice whether the overall tenor of your wardrobe works: If you own a lot of textured, heavy clothing, do you also own chunky shoes and boots to complement them? If you have sexy, silky dresses, skirts, and pants, do you also own a large wardrobe of strappy sandals to complement them? If you own long skirts, do you own stylish, substantial flats to maximize their impact? If you wear miniskirts, do you own adorable flats to complete the look and properly flatter your legs? *Do you own any golden slippers?*

needs

By now, you have spent lots of time editing and assessing your closet—and it's beginning to pay off! You now possess a strong, clear, focused picture of what your wardrobe needs in order to be complete. In terms of shoes, your list may include shoe needs in each category: work, dressy occasions, casual wear, athletic, and sexy. Do your best to record specific details. For example, you don't just need brown shoes for work, sandals for dates, boots for the winter, flats for casual days, gym shoes; you specifically need 3-inch-heeled, burnished brown suede pumps to wear with your tweed skirt; silver metallic sandals to wear with your chiffon dress; winter white suede ankle boots to wear with your favorite winter white cashmere sweater and winter white slacks; brocade flats to spice up your jeans wardrobe; and a pair of orange Stella McCartney athletic shoes to wear to the gym.

I find it is vital to have at least one handbag for each of the ten types of social occasions—very formal, not-so-formal, just-a-teensy-bit formal, informal-but-not-that-informal, every day, every other day, day travel, night travel, theater, and fling.

Miss Piggy

At this time, it's very helpful to distinguish your needs from your wants. "Needs" are shoes that will round out your wardrobe, offer you maximum diversity, complement a minimum of three ensembles, make a declarative fashion statement, enhance your overall appearance, and provide months (or even years) of service. "Wants" are shoes that will add spice to your wardrobe, really dress up an outfit for special occasions, fulfill one of your ultimate fantasies, make your little heart sing every time you put them on, and provide months (or even years) of pleasure.

Begin with your needs, but hold on to and work toward your wants, dreams, and wishes. Once you've rounded out your wardrobe, adopted a brand new *shoe attitude* and *strutted your stuff* down new avenues, you'll deserve a few pairs of dream shoes.

budget

When you're serious about wardrobe building, whether you're dealing with clothes or shoes, you need a plan that includes a carefully crafted fashion budget. It's too easy to fall into the trap of impulse buys, which are usually not so much the items you need as they are the items you fall sway to in a weak moment. Splurging occasionally is something you earn, and the way to win brownie points toward that goal is to create a fashion plan.

Using a spreadsheet format, write down your monthly income in one column and your monthly expenses in another column. Be thorough, making sure to include items like haircuts, cosmetics, entertainment, and Starbucks. Once you have listed every expense you can possibly remember (using your checkbook register helps to make sure you cover everything), earmark 10 percent of your income for savings and allocate a separate amount for emergencies.

What's left is expendable income, which you can then budget for your clothing and footwear needs. Obviously, in revamping, your list of needs probably will be far larger than your expendable income, but with some clever maneuvering, you can maximize value by planning ahead and making smart choices.

priorities

Now that you've established your needs and your budget, it's time to winnow your choices; in other words, prioritize. Go back over your list of needs and rank them according to urgency. Buying the shoes that will most broaden your wardrobe, or buying the shoes that will make a new, definitive statement, makes more sense than buying something with limited use. Despite temptation, it's best to go slowly and stay within your budget. You may feel disheartened, but you'll make far better use of available funds if you create a realistic budget and stick within its parameters.

Also, buy quality over quantity. Part of the *shoe attitude* we've been constructing involves being a smart cookie. When you buy quality products, you're investing in your image the same way you invest in a 401(k). Sure, good shoes are expensive, but you're worth it. Not only will expensive shoes last longer, they'll look fabulous, be far more comfortable than cheap shoes, and they will offer far more fashion bang for the buck. For example, if you pay $200 for a pair of shoes you wear twenty times, that's only $10 per outing. Chances are you'll wear them far more than twenty times, and every time you do, you'll be *strutting your stuff* in style.

But, before you go dashing off to the stores, please review the Appendix in the back of the book for a quick, painless review of Shoes 101 and the art of buying the right size to make your tootsies happy. Go quickly, girls, we're minutes away from sneaking back into your closet to rewrite your footwear fashion profile and totally revitalize your life!

9

change your shoes, change your life—the master plan

Simplicity is the keynote of all true elegance.

now that you've reassessed your wardrobe, you know the holes you need to fill, and you even have a basic game plan in mind. This is where you narrow it down further, refine your goals, and create a master plan for achieving the look you want—allowing, of course, a few wild dreams along the way.

a pair of this, a pair of that
From basic wardrobe to stellar wardrobe

Like our heroine, Cinderella, you've painstak-ingly sorted through your closets and sifted through your past and future dreams, thereby forging a fashion personality. But before you go dashing off to the ball, we'll briefly discuss a bare-bones clothing and shoe wardrobe that will get your life in order, and then quickly move toward a master plan for creating a stellar wardrobe and the life that goes with it.

Bare-bones wardrobes are minimal wardrobes that effectively create and sustain an elegant, workable image. When it comes to bare-bones clothing and shoes, the best course of action involves forsaking trends in favor of classical styling in neutral colors. It's best to select one neutral color to base your entire wardrobe upon, and one coordinating color (black/brown; gray/charcoal; black/navy; forest/olive) through which you can maximize versatility.

bare-bones clothing wardrobe

If you're totally revamping, the basic bare-bones clothing wardrobe consists of the following:

* One black and one white (preferably cashmere) turtleneck
* Several crisp, white blouses
* Two elegant silk blouses
* Several silk sweater sets
* One classically cut black suit
* One knee-length, black sheath dress
* One black and one brown knee-length, pencil skirt
* One pair of black and one pair of brown trousers
* One long, black skirt
* Two pairs of immaculate blue jeans

* One wool coat
* One trench coat
* One leather jacket
* One denim jacket
* One fabulous shawl

bare-bones shoe wardrobe

A bare-bones shoe wardrobe consists of the following classically designed shoes in smooth leathers or suede:

* One pair of black and one pair of brown, mid-heel pumps
* One pair of bone slingbacks
* One pair of black leather knee-high boots
* One pair of black or brown ankle boots
* One pair of brown or black oxfords or loafers
* One pair of evening shoes
* One pair of dressy sandals
* One pair of casual sandals
* One pair of athletic shoes
* Bad-weather boots

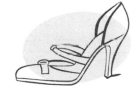

stellar shoe wardrobe

Going from a bare-bones shoe wardrobe to a stellar shoe wardrobe is like going from grammar school in America to graduate school in Europe. Bare-bones wardrobes are a way of creating an image of style and elegance to get by in the world; stellar wardrobes are a way of living, reaching for, and fulfilling your dreams. If you're through with compromising your desires and are determined to live a life that expresses who you are and who you want to be, you're ready for stellar. Stellar shoes are shoes that lift your spirits and mount you to the stars.

You begin by creating an individual style, focusing on details that are distinctive enough to be special, yet classy enough that you will wear them often.

Two courses exist for style creation: broad strokes (heel heights, toe shapes, and silhouette) and details (color, fabrics, patterns, top-stitching, piping, cutouts, and flowerets). Individual style blossoms in the details.

In general, a stellar shoe wardrobe will include all of the bare-bones items, plus the following styles in classic or fringe materials, such as alligator, snakeskin, patent leathers, metallic leathers, velvet, patterned fabrics, and animal prints:

* Ballet flats
* Kitten-heel pumps or slingbacks
* High-heeled (3- to 4-inch) pumps and sandals
* One pair of brown suede knee-high boots
* One pair of red suede boots
* Low-heeled (flat to 1 inch) mules or clogs
* Metallic sandals
* Rhinestone sandals
* Snakeskin sandals
* Flat thong sandals
* Alligator pumps or boots

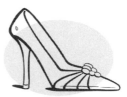

color

Red is the great clarifier—bright, cleansing, and revealing. It makes all the other colors beautiful. I can't imagine becoming bored with red; it would be like becoming bored with the person you love.

Diana Vreeland

Color takes a shoe from basic to standout, from serviceable to pleasurable, from tasteful to defining. Color packs emotional wallop, plus nourishes your spirit *and* uplifts your entire wardrobe. When it comes to color, consider shaking the rafters occasionally. Here's some basic information on color delineations to prime your color wheel:

* Subdued = black (backdrop color)
* Neutral colors = gray, tan, navy, brown
* Pastels = pale pink, light green, baby blue
* Brights = electric blue, lime, orange, yellow, green
* Mid-tones = melon, deep lavender, rose (saturated pastels)
* Jewel tones = emerald, sapphire, ruby
* Warm colors = chocolates, brick, eggplant, forest green

Colors also carry an emotional quotient that can be personal or universal. The reason so many men wear black suits is that black is almost universally associated with authority or power. *A la* Audrey Hepburn, many women associate black with classic chic. These universal associations may or may not be how you relate to a color. For instance, when it comes to clothing, some people consider head-to-toe black so overpowering it makes them look washed out or drained of their power. When it comes to choosing your favorite shoe colors, the following universal emotional quotients can serve as a springboard to help you define your personal preferences. In shoes, for example, black is always classic, but to you it may feel more like a standard-bearer; maybe your shoe power color is purple.

* Black = always classic, always chic, a power color
* Brown = earthy, classic, denotes stability, old money
* Burgundy, plum, forest, charcoal, navy = dark neutrals, alternatives to black
* Light gray = classic Grace Kelly, the new summer white
* Beige/cream/camel/taupe = timeless chic, far superior to white
* Winter white = acceptable in winter boots
* White = only when you're wearing white; best limited to summer sandals
* Red = vital, energetic, powerful, successful, sexually appealing
* Pink = feminine, subtly sexy, healthy, glowing
* Green = rebirth, renewal, spring, growth
* Blue = peace, tranquility, spirituality
* Purple = royalty, vibrancy, richness
* Yellow = joyful, playful, sunny
* Orange = lively, happy, friendly, earthy when subtle

* **Color Do:** When it's time to mix and match, remember that Mother Nature embraces a myriad of color combinations: green with purple, pink, lavender, or yellow; beige with heathers, greens, blues, and charcoal.
* **Color Do:** Warm tones of copper or bronze and cooler tones of dulled silver, pewter, or gray are stylish neutral alternatives.

* **Color Don't:** Stark white pumps make your feet look bigger and your taste questionable. For a classier alternative, wear bone, taupe, tan, pastels, or subdued metallic leathers.
* **Big Color Don't:** "Avoid colors that remind you of an airport in Florida." Anna Johnson, author of *Three Black Skirts*

Hint: Matching your shoes to your hair color and skin tones creates a very polished look and elongates your overall image.

it's in the details

Other ways to catapult your shoe wardrobe from bares bones to stellar is to spice up your shoes through details, including:

* **Trim:** piping, cutouts, perforations, strapping, embroidery, appliques, and beading.
* **Texture:** multiple tones, multiple leathers, fabric, suede, alligator, etc.
* **Embellishments:** metal ornaments, buttons, buckles, bows, rhinestones pasted onto fabric or straps, paste-on or clip-on ornaments (*hint*: try flowered hair clips), rhinestones pasted onto heels.

Finally, make a list of things you love—sensuality, taste, colors, sounds, textures, styles—and then give them credence by finding clever ways to incorporate these passions into your game plan. Kirsten Amann, assistant editor for an East Coast publishing firm, had a passion for art and realized upon revamping her closet that she didn't have any outrageous, personal-expression shoes in her collection. When shopping one day, she found a pair of somewhat funky open-toed shoes made out of an eclectic combination of navy blue leather, deep blue denim, and cream-colored fabric dotted with precious little red rosettes on a very high, wood heel. "I thought they were dreamy, but a real stretch, both in terms of my shoe budget and my personal expression. What would I wear them with? They were so odd—still, I fell in love with them and wanted them desperately. When I took them home, I soon became very creative in pairing them with outfits. So far I've worn them with my vintage-y black strapless dress that has an A-line skirt reminiscent of the fifties; with my mid-length blue cropped pants and a light summer sweater for casual Friday at the office; and with my boot-cut designer jeans and a sparkly top for evening cocktails. Not only did I learn that I'm far better at mixing and matching than I originally thought; every time I wear my fabulous, funky shoes they bring out—and show the world—my more artistic side."

a shoe for all seasons

Shoe shopping to meet your goals, overcome your obstacles, and fulfill your dreams

Trends are general, gentle shifts in shape and mood. A trend in footwear would include a movement toward narrow silhouettes, more rounded toes, knee-high boots, or romantic fabrications. Fads, on the other hand, are hot looks that fade quickly—garish prints or colors, scuffed-up Frye boots, metallic leathers studded

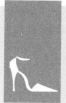

designer dish

Miuccia Prada

WONDER WOMAN

The Prada family founded their shoe factory in 1923, and although always known for the creation of expensive, high-quality footwear, it wasn't until Miuccia took the helm in the late 1970s that they became fashion innovators. Every shoe became a bold fashion statement, reflecting the personality of the wearer, offering extreme luxury and creative whimsy. Memorable shoes: Silver Screen Goddess shoes with chunky gold heels and art déco styling. Patrons include today's most dedicated followers of fashion.

with oversized rhinestones, flimsy flip-flops, Chinese slippers for street wear, or white patent go-go boots.

To maximize wear, build your stellar wardrobe around timeless shoes. Timeless shoes usually have simple lines, no frills or low frills, and quality materials and craftsmanship. Timeless shoes look great in a multitude of situations.

Also, a general rule of thumb is that you don't need more; you need better. Singular excellence *always* trumps quantity; one perfect shoe is worth five mediocre shoes. Expensive shoes buy a lot of chic and provide long-term fashion mileage. Manolo Blahnik, for example, designs far more timeless styles than trendy styles, making the cost of his shoes a true fashion investment. To build a strong shoe wardrobe, buy versatile, classic, neutral-colored shoes, and then add intelligently and slowly. Once you have established a shoe wardrobe that meets your needs, spending money on exotic, fashion shoes adds the necessary spice and vigor that rounds out your image and makes life fun.

creating a wish book

Because magazines and advertising agencies hire top professional stylists to style advertisements and editorial illustrations, you can take advantage of their expertise to maximize your makeover. Buy yourself a stack of fashion magazines—European magazines frequently are fabulous sources of preseason information—to determine fashion trends, what works with what, what would or would not work for you, what you love or hate, what makes sense or doesn't make sense, what you crave. What you see in magazines usually reflects the most expensive fashion choices out there, but you can duplicate or draw from these looks to bolster your wardrobe.

When I was a little girl, my sisters and I would eagerly await the Sears Roebuck catalog, which everyone called the *"wish book."*

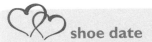 **shoe date**

Invite three of your best girlfriends over for a Sunday brunch. Introduce them to the *wish book* philosophy. Ask each to bring fashion magazines (definitely include European ones!) and a journal. Serve a light brunch, including mimosas, and then gather in a circle to select shoes and outfits from the magazines. You may be surprised (and delighted) to discover what your friends suggest for you, and vice versa. Cheers!

When it arrived, we spent hours flipping through its pages, carefully selecting outfits we longed to have. Months later, when my mother would finally surrender the catalog, my sister and I would cut out our favorite people and create our wished-for lives, based almost solely on the wardrobes that our cutouts were wearing. We would keep these images in shoeboxes in our closet, pulling them out often to pretend we were living the life we dreamed they had.

Okay, it's hokey, but it taught me to dream, and to envision a life bigger than the one I was living. By pasting pictures in a *wish book*, you are deeply envisioning the image you want to create, which will not only help you actually achieve a real makeover, but also will save you thousands of dollars in misspent funds. I recommend leafing through all your magazines first, and then going back to retrieve images. Keep in mind your overall fashion personality, but also keep in mind the various archetypes, exploring new avenues you might want to embrace. Pretend you're a costume designer who is searching for images of clothing, footwear, accessories, colors, textures, and lifestyle that would create an exciting, accurate image for your subject.

Reality is a world as you feel it to be, as you wish it to be, as you wish it into being.

Diana Vreeland

Let's say that you're interested in spicing up your work wardrobe. Perhaps you'll see a photograph of a woman wearing a pink Chanel jacket with a pair of jeans in one ad; a woman wearing a pink-and-brown-striped silk blouse in another; a woman wearing a chocolate-brown suede pencil skirt in another; a woman wearing a pair of

shoe do

Before you rush out the door to buy new shoes, take a moment to learn an appreciation for high-quality footwear. Pull out your most expensive shoes, and look for the following tell-all signs of workmanship:

- Excellent design
- Great fit qualities
- Top-grade materials
- Leather lining, leather sole
- Superior workmanship, uniform stitching
- Strong silhouette
- Aspect of timelessness

On your shopping excursions, keep these characteristics in mind when making your purchasing decisions.

brown suede pumps with pink piping in another; and a woman wearing a brown butterfly brooch in another. Paste all of these images together on one page, *et voilà*, you've created a fresh look for the office. While you may not hunt down the exact pieces, you have created an image map of what you're looking for.

Once you have a stack of images, pair them with compatible images. To begin, separate the images into categories: work, date, casual, dressy, workout, etc. Take one pile at a time and play mix and match. Group images according to what you want to coordinate—textures, colors, styles—arranging them in inventive ways to refine the look even further, honing it down to specific blouses, sweaters, handbags, and shoes that will compile your final image.

When you have images assembled, paste them into the appropriate sections of your *wish book*. Leave several pages next to each grouping blank so that you can denote specific details, colors, or matching items you either already possess or want to find. If you already have three outfits in your wardrobe that you can pair with a particular pair of shoes, list the outfits so you'll have them in mind when you're shopping. If the picture is close but not exactly what you want, write down what you want: "similar look on a 2-inch heel"; "strappy sandal in gold metallic." Keep in mind that it isn't necessary to buy the actual shoe in the picture; you are using the photograph as a guide to find shoes that duplicate the look by imitating shapes, colors, details, and proportions (heel height, toe shape, platform height, etc.).

The hope is that you'll not only find this exercise relaxing and highly enjoyable, but extremely productive in terms of building an image. Ideally, you'll update your fashion *wish book* at least twice a year—preferably four times a year—and develop an unshakable habit of taking it with you when you shop.

 need some shoe inspiration?

Check out these fabulous Internet sites, and you'll be on the way to your stellar shoe wardrobe in no time:

Style.com	*Luckymag.com*	*Bizrate.com*
Instyle.com	*Mightyflirt.com*	*Mysimon.com*
Fashionfinds.com	*Eluxury.com*	*More-shoes.com*
Fashiondish.com	*Niemanmarcus.com*	*Onlineshoes.com*
Net-a-porter.com	*Nordstrom.com*	*Shoemall.com*
Katespade.com	*Footcandy.com*	*Macys.com*

on your mark . . . get set . . . shop!

Prior to hitting the stores, it's important to broaden your perspective and sharpen your shopping skills. Researching Internet sites is a great way to learn about trends, product, and prices. A list of sites featuring overall fashion trends follows, along with several department store sites (Neiman Marcus, Nordstrom, and Macy's are fabulous shoe resources). You also can use a search engine (Yahoo or Google, for example) to locate Web sites for local stores and designers, many of whom feature their biographies and their latest collections. By spending time canvassing these sites, you familiarize yourself with current trends in clothing, footwear, and accessories. You also will be able to pinpoint designs that meet your needs and either go right to the source or find resources for duplicating the look in a less expensive brand. This is time well spent; you'll gain invaluable knowledge of the market that will help you make wise choices when in the trenches. The more you learn about fashion, and the more you learn about yourself—or your emerging self—the better you'll become at maximizing your fashion budget dollars.

ten commandments of shopping

Okay, now that you're *finally* ready to shop, let's discuss ten shopping commandments that will make you a pro, obtain the desired results, and maximize your fashion expenditures.

1. Do your homework first.

Your *wish book* should be full of holes you need to fill—in clothing, shoes, handbags, and accessories. Between the *shoe dos* and *shoe*

precious cargo

In the 1990s, Manolo Blahnik created 18-karat-gold sandals valued at $12,000 a pair for an Antonio Berardi fashion show. Because burglars stole merchandise from his previous collection, Berardi not only hired bodyguards to protect the shoes, he made sure someone counted the shoes as they went on and came off the models' feet, never allowing the shoes out of sight.

dates and heeding my advice, hopefully, you have researched Web sites and shopped in several department stores, as well as two of the best shoe stores in your area. The Internet shopping will acquaint you with the variety of options on the market and train your eye toward current trends. If you see items you particularly love or items that fit perfectly into your plan, print the pictures and paste them into your *wish book*. Visit several large department stores on an exploratory shopping venture—not buying, only looking. Again, be an archeologist and determine current styles, trends, colors, details, and so on. Feel free to try on twenty-five pairs, but do not buy anything. Try on the most expensive shoes in each department; so you'll know what it feels like to have the best. Notice how the leather molds to your feet, how the heel is balanced, and how comfortable a well-made, well-constructed, well-executed shoe feels. Notice all the nuances, the suppleness of the leather, the leather lining, the way leather breathes. Take your digital camera and ask the clerk if you can photograph certain styles—so you can come back for them. If you can't do that, jot down details and place the photograph or the list of details in your *wish book* for future reference.

2. Never go shopping without your wish book.

You may think you'll remember what's on your "must-buy" list, but think about all those times you've stood in a grocery store aisle trying desperately to remember what you rushed to the store to buy. It's even more difficult to remember what you need in clothing and shoes. Your memory may not serve you well, and all your careful preparation can go out the window. You worked to create a concrete plan for building an overall image; going shopping without your *wish book* may lead to piecemeal buying, which defeats your ultimate purpose.

3. Shop alone.

While it's always fun to shop with girlfriends, save those occasions for splurge buying. Exploratory shopping and serious shopping require maximum concentration. With girlfriends, it's too easy to lose your focus, surrender your best intentions, and succumb to (unconscious) peer pressure—you're more likely to order dessert if your girlfriend does. Spending hundreds of dollars on shoes is an investment; would you make an investment decision in the middle of a conversation? When you've taken the time and energy to do your homework, you don't require your girlfriend's opinion. Of course, great merit exists in comparison shopping or scouting missions with girlfriends. Take your *wish book* along, write down the items you want to consider, and, if you wake up two days later convinced those shoes were perfect, run back to the store and purchase them.

4. Ask for help.

Particularly in high-quality department stores, specialty retailers, or high-end boutiques, salesclerks know their inventory and

using descriptive words to justify new shoes

About to swipe that credit card and feeling twinges of hesitation? Worried about what your boyfriend, husband, best friend, or teenage daughter will say when you come home with yet another pair of fabulous shoes? Try these justifications on for size. They're guaranteed to dispel your doubts, leave you feeling footloose and fancy-free, and silence your critics:

- They're surrealistic.
- They're baroque.
- They're modernist.
- They're flamboyant.
- They're so minimalist.
- They make me feel like a seductress.
- When I wear them, I feel competitive.
- When I wear them, I feel like a pit bull.
- They brand me.
- They're sophisticated.
- They're supremely romantic.
- They're real attention-getters.
- They've very understated.
- They're funky.
- They're couture, darling.
- They celebrate culture.
- They're my power shoes.
- They're my sexy shoes.

- They're my after-eight shoes.
- These are my life-event shoes.
- They're the ultimate ensemble shoes.
- They have the right logo.
- They represent the crème de la crème.
- They're living art.
- They provide a serious material function.
- They're vintage treasures.
- They are timeless investments.
- These are thrift-shop jewels.
- They create mystery.
- They add to my mystique.
- They provided shameless retail therapy.
- They give me fashion credibility.
- They'll be my constant companions.

their business, meaning they will have excellent style, fit, and price recommendations. If you don't ask for help, you may miss an opportunity to upgrade or find the best shoe for the best price. If you have problem feet, go to stores that specialize in comfort footwear and ask for their most experienced salesperson. You deserve the best!

Luxury is the necessity that begins where necessity ends.
Coco Chanel

5. Buy shoes that fit in your plan first.

Until you have your basics covered, avoid trend and impulse buys. The most important thing you want to do is to build a solid, classic wardrobe. If you have dispensable funds to blow, go for it. If not, buy on program.

6. If they don't fit, they don't go home.

No arguments. Stretching, easing, and wearing-in do little to alter the way the shoes will fit. If your feet hurt, you'll never look good—period. Even Oprah, an admitted shoe fanatic, traditionally wears what she calls "one-hour shoes" for her shows and occasionally wears "two-minute shoes," meaning they are slipped off her feet as soon as she sits down. Oprah can afford this luxury; the rest of us must be a teensy bit more prudent.

7. Avoid retrograde.

No resorting to tried and true; no reliving the past. You are buying shoes for the new you, not the old you. Reinterpretations of bygone eras are over.

8. Buy the most expensive shoes you can afford.

You are far better off streamlining your wardrobe and owning a few pairs of expensive, high-quality shoes than owning a closetful of inexpensive, lackluster shoes that won't wear well or long.

9. If you can't afford them, restrain yourself.

Exception: If they are within the top three priorities in your *wish book* and you can visualize six outfits they will immediately complement, consider using your credit card. If they don't meet the above criteria, pull out your *wish book*, pore over your list, and reconsider long and hard. Sleep on it, and, if you still hunger for them the next day . . . well, fine.

10. If you absolutely love them, throw caution to the wind.

In other words, if they are so totally you or totally who you want to be that just holding them in your hands stirs a visceral reaction, akin to love at first sight, buy them. Note: You must be absolutely wild about them, and you must have enough money left over to pay rent and buy food for a month.

trend spotting

A guide to bargain shopping

Obviously, the majority of us cannot afford top designer labels, nor would many of us consider them remotely essential. Designers are fabulous resources for fashion direction—silhouette, style, color, heel height, toe shape, textures, etc. Use them as inspiration. Like all manufacturers, shoe factories notoriously copy designs.

By applying your resources—actually applying shoe leather by window-shopping expensive, trendsetting stores in your area to predetermine what you want to find at a lower price point, conducting Internet and magazine research, and creating your *wish book*—you'll find ways to easily replicate designer fashions at far more affordable price points.

Two-thirds of all women buy trends on sale—good girls! Other ways to bargain shop include the following:

✳ Stick to your plan!
✳ Shop around before buying; save up for special purchases.
✳ For inside information, make friends with salesclerks. Find out when they execute markdowns; frequently, department store

 footwear follies

- In 1998, Judy Garland's *Wizard of Oz* ruby slippers fetched $187,000.
- Another pair of Judy Garland's shoes, designed by shoemaker to the stars (and my wedding shoes creator!) Pasquale Di Fabrizio, sold for $126,000 at auction.
- Beverly Hills jeweler Harry Winston, "The King of Diamonds," pavéd 4,500 rubies on a pair of pumps to duplicate the ruby slippers.
- Ruby-colored rhinestone Salvatore Ferragamo pumps once owned by Marilyn Monroe sold for $48,300 at a 1999 Christie's auction.
- Gina's of London won an entry in the Guinness Book of World Records for creating the most expensive shoes in history. Her slim handcrafted snakeskin, high-heeled mules featuring white gold buckles inlaid with thirty-six princess-cut diamonds were valued at $25,000 a pair.

managers meet every Monday to assign markdowns that show up on the floor Tuesday. You also can get the inside track on progressive markdowns simply by asking for their schedule. Also, get the facts on their markdown policy; often, if you buy a pair of shoes that go on sale one or even two weeks later, you can return with your receipt for credit.

* To get first dibs and avoid weekend sale crowds, hit the stores late Friday night.

* Never buy anything you can't wear with at least three, and preferably five, outfits.

* Allow yourself an occasional splurge (it's like starving yourself and then eating five chocolate truffles because you feel so deprived). Indulging occasionally helps prevent disastrous overspending.

* Remember that fads are usually over by the time they're on sale (it's okay to buy them if you're ahead of the curve, if they're made of fabric, or if they're marked way, way down). *Hint*: make your own fads instead!

* Buy classics and workhorses on sale. Who thought Hush Puppies would make a return? (Ditto Burberry trench coats, preppy clothing, black everything.) Athletic shoes, classic black pumps, classic black boots, splendid, timeless dress sandals—if you love them—all make good buys when spotted with a great markdown.

* Buy the really expensive items off-season, when they're on sale. Buy boots in January (or better yet, February); buy strappy dress sandals in fall or after the holiday season.

* Summer shoes are less expensive and generally have the shortest season; buy inexpensive sandals and save your bucks for fall.

* If you live near a major metropolitan area, check your newspapers for sample sale listings.
* Haunt renowned discount stores like Marshall's and Loehmann's; both are famous for an ever-revolving, fabulously discounted inventory of shoe treasures.

curbing binges

Making smart choices without succumbing to shoe addiction

In Paris, shopping is a serious interval in one's life—perhaps twice a year. It's a pilgrimage.

Diana Vreeland

One of the major differences between Parisian women and American women is that Parisian women own far fewer clothes and shoes. Their stores reflect their lifestyle: expensive, fabulously stylish, high-quality merchandise in small quantities. Parisian women have an innate confidence that helps them greatly when it comes to assembling edited wardrobes that reflect everything they want to reflect, including their refined sense of taste. They don't feel compelled, as so many Americans do, to stuff their closets; instead, they carefully select a few outfits and wear them repeatedly over the course of several years. They are not nomadic shoppers, nor are they compulsive shoppers.

In fact, excessive shopping can be a monumental waste of creative energy. It becomes addictive when you constantly feel compelled to spend, as if doing so will fill the holes in your life. One clue that you're addicted: the high you feel lasts less than twenty minutes. If you have problems with compulsive shopping, make a list of other activities that make you feel good, focusing on ones that make you feel good about yourself as opposed to those that deliver a temporary high, and pursue one of them whenever the urge to shop arises. Do this steadily and you'll find that other activities fulfill your emotional needs far better than mindless shopping does.

When an urge to shop unnecessarily arises—say, when your budget is squat and you don't really, *really* need anything—stall long enough to rate your urge to shop. Is the urge arising from a legitimate but low-priority need, a precocious want, a desire to stem boredom, or a desire to boost flagging self-esteem? If you're still selling yourself on the idea, retrieve your *wish book* and review your goals to determine whether you have a real need.

If you don't, divert your urge to shop and funnel the energy into revamping your closet. If you imagine that your closet is a small, exclusive boutique and pull out new style combinations, you can have as much fun shopping your closet as you would shopping the mall. Go full tilt: lay out jewelry, belts, handbags, and scarves, and then spend hours playing mix and match. When you find new combinations, write them down so you'll remember to weave them into your ongoing wardrobe. This also is a good time to work on regular maintenance, pulling items that need cleaning or mending.

If you remain determined to go shopping, eat a healthy meal and dress up so you'll leave feeling satisfied *and* good about yourself. Before you leave your house, review your *wish book* and make a short list of items you are willing to buy. Predetermine the amount you can afford to spend and then withdraw it from an ATM. When your cash is gone, you're done.

If these methods haven't dimmed your burning desire to shop, consider the following quote:

There's times when I just have to quit thinking . . . and the only way I can quit thinking is by shopping.
                                    Tammy Faye (Bakker) Messner

We're all smart girls, aren't we? We value ourselves, *and* we value thinking.

Now that we've covered all the basics, forged a fashion personality, created a *wish book*, examined our motives, and geared up for ultra-smart shopping, it's time to wrap up this party. In the next chapter, we'll cover tips and techniques and offer up outrageous ideas for celebrating your shoe obsession. Hurry, girls, your prince is waiting.

10

the future's so bright, i gotta wear new shoes

Fashion is the most fickle of muses, but it is her very capriciousness which has captivated and inspired men. If she is one thing today, tomorrow she will be another.

Anna Harvey, <u>British Vogue</u>

throughout this journey together, you've been transitioning from the woman you were to the woman you want to be. You've been in the process of *being and becoming*, which means you have cast off the chains of an unexamined life and embraced the benefits of a chosen, self-directed, evolving one. By examining how your wardrobe reflects how you think, act, and walk through your life and taking all the steps to create and live the image you desire, you have effectively removed the wooden shoes of your past and donned your golden slippers. *Being and becoming* is where you'll want to remain—

immediately recognizing boredom or ineffectiveness, evaluating, assessing, and redefining your choices, and transitioning into a newer, expanded vision of yourself. Now that you've learned the value of constantly reassessing your lifestyle, you're well on your way to creating your own, distinct *shoe attitude.* Before we send you off to *strut your stuff,* it's time for fine-tuning.

tips and tricks

For the dance scene in *Funny Face,* the director wanted Audrey Hepburn to wear white socks to contrast with her black dance out-fit. Audrey was livid; she insisted the white socks interrupted the flow of her outfit and made her legs look shorter. Audrey wasn't just being persnickety; she understood the subtle art of fine-tuning. As such, the following advice from fashion experts will help you fine-tune your *shoe attitude.*

Basics

* Wardrobes need rotation.
* Great shoes elevate your entire outfit.
* Chic means assimilating the best elements of a new fashion season or selecting one or two trendy items and using them to refresh, but not violate, your sense of style.
* Every time you make a new purchase, take time to assemble outfits and write them down so you'll remember to incorporate them into your wardrobe rotation.
* Avoid anything that screams "I'm still young."
* Colored shoes add real punch to a monochromatic outfit.

The Skinny on Fat and Skinny

Certain styles flatter certain figures. If you are a larger woman, wearing thinly heeled shoes can make you look heavier; whereas a woman with very thin legs will look even thinner if she wears chunky shoes. The following suggestions are designed to help you maximize your body type and achieve a slenderizing, pulled-together look.

* Wearing matching opaque stockings with boots elongates your leg.
* Midcalf boots cut your leg in half right at its fattest part (boots look best when they taper at the ankle and fit your calf snugly).
* Skinny calves only look twiggier on chunky shoes or thick heels.
* Big calves only look bigger on skinny shoes and thin or kitten heels.
* High vamps shorten the appearance of your legs (but look fabulous with pants).
* Thick T-straps shorten your foot (a good thing) and your leg (not so good). Men love them despite this, so occasional wear for specific purposes is still advised. If you've got great legs, thin T-straps provide a classic look.
* Open-toed sandals elongate your legs right down to your toes. Thinly strapped or flesh-colored sandals slim even more.
* Crisscross straps trim down plump ankles (particularly if the straps are midfoot and thin).
* Narrow straps are slimming; thick straps are fattening.
* Petites need shoes that elongate their feet—low vamps, pointed toes, and 2- to 3-inch sculpted heels work great; avoid chunky heels or wedges.
* Low-cut vamps and slingbacks are slimming.

how to rate your morning after . . .

According to *The Bad Girl's Guide to the Party Life* by Cameron Tuttle.

Buzz Kill: passing out in your hostess' closet

Buzz Thrill: waking up at home the next morning wearing new Prada shoes

Mix and Match

Even though a woman with *shoe attitude* reserves the right to break all the rules, certain styles of shoes generally do look best when paired with certain clothing. Consider the following guidelines, then create your own exceptions.

∗   When wearing particularly dressy clothes, the simpler your shoe, the better.

∗   If you are wearing a multicolored skirt, dress, or pants, match shoe and hosiery color tones to the color closest to the hemline.

∗   The shorter the skirt, the flatter the shoe.

∗   Narrow pants look best with low heels.

∗   Heavily textured and bulky clothing look best with heavier shoes.

∗   Long skirts look best with low-heeled, sleek shoes or sandals. High boots in a similar tonal range also work well.

∗   Platforms with short skirts make heavier legs look heavier and skinny legs look skinnier. Limit platforms to pants or long skirts.

And Finally . . .

Think of your closet as your favorite high-scale, specialized boutique, and shop it regularly!

playing dress-up

As soon as I discovered, in a cardboard box in the attic, Mother's old sorority-girl crêpe-de-chine evening dresses in shades of apricot, marigold, and avocado green, I was hooked on glamour . . . Their delicately beaded bodices and slim-fitting, bias-cut skirts pinned tightly over my stick-like body triggered a clothes meme in my DNA and I became Greta Garbo.

Melissa Hook, in an essay entitled <u>Material Girl</u>

Remember how much fun you had playing dress-up as a child? That's because you were literally trying on various personas, feeling the energy of being a princess, a movie star, a mother, a teacher, a firefighter. As you slipped the crinolines over your head and retrieved those little pink mules on rubber kitten heels from the coveted place in your closet, you assembled the *accoutrements* and the personality of a princess. Remember strutting around the room in the kitten heels, balancing a tiara on your head, fluffing the folds of your pink satin princess dress, and lifting its hem as you mounted the imaginary stairs to your castle? This may have been your first taste of how it feels to simply be born special, and, if you were lucky, you transformed this game of pretend into viable *shoe attitude*. Maybe the next time you walked through the grammar school cafeteria, you assumed the princess attitude and your demeanor commanded attention. Maybe the next time a boy looked your way, you thrust your shoulders back, lifted your chin, exuded confidence, and knew you landed him in your stable of potential admirers.

The benefits of playing dress-up didn't have to end with childhood. We all play a form of dress-up when we shop for new clothes or shoes, or when frantically searching for an outfit to wear for a special occasion. Those forms of dress-up are valid, but all too frequently we don't *really* get into the game. Instead, we select familiar items in familiar combinations. Playing dress-up in a way that benefits *shoe attitude* requires leaps into fantasy.

As you stretch your own boundaries and add depth to your wardrobe and your *shoe attitude*, play dress-up for real. When it's time for the next party, why not pick some of your more adventurous clothing and shoes? If you're like me, you store "special items" in the back of your closet to wait (and wait and wait) for the right occasion to break them out. Well, girls, no more waiting! Pull those special items out and try them on. Try them on with all your other special items—the antique lace shawl you found in Italy, your grandmother's diamond brooch, the flapper hat you found in your attic when you were a child, the 3-inch, hand-tooled sterling cuff bracelets you bought on a trip to Arizona—in unique and adventurous possibilities. Pretend you are Carolina Herrera, Stevie Nicks, Carrie Bradshaw, or Beyoncé.

When in doubt, overdress.
Vivienne Westwood

One of my more adventurous, strong-minded, self-motivated, dynamic friends buys long, black lace formfitting dresses; saucy, oversized red bonnets; and red stiletto T-straps that I would consider suitable for a hot date—and wears them when we go out for Sunday brunch in Sacramento. While I am always adequately dressed, for example, in a cute knee-length, denim skirt, paired with a twinset and low-heeled sandals, this friend buys outrageous clothes and shoes and then plays dress-up every day! She not only lives the life she wants, she has infinitely more fun than most people do.

My daughter, Brooke, is the same way. When she buys a sexy T-shirt with a gauze overlay or a pair of platform sandals bedazzled with rhinestones, she wears them the very next day—no matter where she's going. "I'm interested in dressing to be the best Brooke I can be. Unless it's me, I don't even buy it. And if it's me, then I want it to be me right now, today, not tomorrow, and not maybe next week. Why wait?"

Why indeed? If you're not playing dress-up, you're not creating opportunities to expand your personality, surprise your friends, wake up your lovers, and make your bosses do a double take. Worse than that, if you're not creating opportunities to explore, what are you waiting for?

 shoe do

When shopping, wander in and through clothing, shoe, and accessory departments you normally miss—designer, young, evening, professional suiting, sports. As you peruse their wares, pull items that you normally would pass by and simply try them on—try, really try, to surprise yourself. In doing so, you may loosen self-imposed strictures and discover a piece of your personality that was long hidden or buried. You may discover that donning a pair of Manolo Blahniks makes you feel like Grace Kelly or the Princess of Moravia. You may discover that donning a pair of Ralph Lauren equestrian boots makes you feel like a warrior goddess or the owner of Montana horse ranch. You may discover that donning a pair of Christian Louboutin satin pumps makes you feel like Kate Hudson on a hot date, or a sexy woman in her prime.

experimentation

Taking chances and walking on the wild side

Remember that art frequently results from disharmony; never be afraid to shake things up occasionally. I'm not suggesting you break all the rules, even though a woman with *shoe attitude* possesses the knowledge and courage required to break a few rules occasionally.

 shoe date: let's have a shoe party!

Okay, we love our shoes and our shoes love us. Now that we've done all the homework and taken our shoe conversion very seriously, it's time to break out some champagne and have a little wicked fun. Why not call your shoe-loving girlfriends together for a playful evening? Fresh out of ideas? Give these a shot.

Costume Party   Create a theme—*sneaker down, pump up, gladiator goddess, rhinestone cowgirl, hooker harlot, or divine diva*—and then invite your friends to dress up in full costume. Have each friend bring an appropriate theme song, and have fun dancing around the room acting like goddesses, gladiators, cowgirls, or divas!

Fantasy Land   Have friends bring over a box of costume items (boas, tiaras, pink rhinestone sandals, beaded shawls, fur stoles, rhinestone hair clips, brooches the size of Texas, angel wings) and then spend the night playing dress-up. Let girlfriends have a turn at putting you together, and then parade your new personality around the room to see if any of its elements fit the new you.

Matchmaker   Invite friends to bring over their most challenging mix-and-match items. Throw everything into a pile and spend the evening playing *what goes with what*.

I'm suggesting that you experiment occasionally by mixing a classic suit with an avant-garde pair of shoes, or sexy, filmy skirt with chunky boots. It's simply fun to surprise everyone, including you. The following are a few suggestions to get your creativity engine revved up.

* Wear your sexiest dressy sandals with your favorite jeans, topped with a furry jacket, glitzy drop earrings, and a funky handbag.
* Wear your classic little black dress with green suede boots, dangling gypsy earrings, and a green fringed shawl.
* Wear your tailored black suit with wildly colored fabric pumps.
* Wear your sexiest flower-patterned voile flirty skirt with your scuffed cowboy boots, a raggedy jeans jacket, a cowboy belt, and a Hermès watch.
* Wear your most expensive, classic shoes with edgy outfits to create your own style.

incorporating accessories

Matching accessories is so mother-of-the-bride.
Anna Johnson, author of Three Black Skirts

While shoes are your primary accessory, cunning selection and inventiveness is key when it comes to completing your look. Accessories, and accessory coordination, are your best shot at achieving individuality. Obviously, you want them to work well together, to complement your silhouette and your wardrobe, but the manner in which you assemble the total package is where your individuality lies. Mixing and matching contemporary shoes, shawls, belts, scarves, handbags, and jewelry can take you from vintage to contemporary, from classic to bohemian, from romantic to business—and back again.

Clothes without accessories are like sex without orgasm.
Robert Lee Morris, jewelry designer

Just remember: Your clothes and shoes are the stars; your accessories the supporting actors. Accessories support, complement, enhance, and define your wardrobe. Although it's important to fine-tune socks, bags, belts, hosiery, jewelry, sweaters, and scarves, focus on creating one star and allow the rest to be supporting players.

First, let's examine what we expect accessories to do:

Enhance Your Clothing and Shoes

Choose accessories that draw out the accents in your outfit:

* A suede jacket that matches the piping on your suede pumps
* A contemporary pearl necklace that mirrors the trim on your beaded evening shoes
* A chain belt that duplicates the chain detailing on your shoes and handbag

Create a Very Pulled-Together Look

While you don't want to appear as if you work at it, the selection of intentionally coordinating accessories lets the world know that you know what you're doing. Examples include the following.

* Black dress, multicolored beaded shawl, and similarly styled, multicolored beaded sandals
* Matching brown alligator shoes, handbag, and watch strap
* Navy suede fringed boots with navy suede fringed jacket

Make a Serious Style Statement

Far too often we settle for what looks good together when we could actually choose one or two accessories that make a bold fashion statement, taking us from passable to sensational. Consider wearing:

* Crisp white blouse, denim culottes, and riding boots topped with an aqua cashmere shawl
* Green suede dress paired with feathered shoes, handbag, and hat

Add Drama

Why not shake up your world and everyone around you occasionally? It's simply great fun to play a dramatic role once in a while. Often, a single accessory achieves it, such as:

* An oversized, boldly colored picture hat with plain sheath dress
* A purple velvet cloche hat with a long black wool dress
* A veiled hat with a daytime satin suit

Jewelry isn't meant to make you look rich, it's meant to adorn you, and that is not the same thing.

Coco Chanel

Maximize Your Assets

As you accumulate accessories, view them as ways to maximize your fashion quotient and think long-term investment. To maximize accessories, you'll want to follow a few basic tenets, such as:

* **Create a fluid balance.** If your wardrobe is overstocked in one particular category, at the expense of all the others, it throws your budget and your fashion image out-of-balance. What's the point of having twenty-five handbags if you only have three pairs of shoes?

* **Buy quality over quantity!** I've said it before and I'll say it again: You're *always* better off buying a few high-quality items than a plethora of inexpensive items! The cheap ones will show their wear within months, and besides, this is *you* we're talking about, and you deserve the best!

* **Buy current. You'll want to** to look *au courant*, not trendy, lest you risk undermining your long-term fashion image. Obviously you want to keep up-to-date, but purchasing one pair of pumps and a matching handbag in this season's color and shape will update your image without breaking the bank.

* **Be on trend without being trendy.** Trendy has its place in your closet, but buying one hot new handbag, a few pairs of fashionable earrings, or two hair accessories keeps you in the fashion game without blowing your budget on something that won't be in style next season.

* **Don't forget day-to-day flair**—it will individualize your style and put your personal stamp on every outfit. If you're famous for wearing scarves, splurge on a few fabulous newcomers.

Once you amass a wardrobe of accessories, you can increase your fashion quotient by subtly, or boldly, coordinating accessories to take you from boring to fabulous. Consider the following:

Scale Is Important

If you're wearing a pair of spaghetti-strapped sandals teetering on a thin high heel, a jumbo tote will throw you off balance—literally and visually. On the other hand (or foot), a bulky sweater and long wool skirt paired with a pair of thick-soled boots and a suede tote would work well. Basically, coordinate the proportion of your accessories, and you'll balance the scales in your favor.

Color Coordinate

Color/tonal mixing works best when all of your accessories are in the same tonal range. Obvious *faux pas* include dark stockings with white shoes or vice versa (ouch, so obviously hideous). While it's fun to play with colors—and we do want to have fun—if your shoes, handbag, scarves, hats, and gloves are in a coordinating color or at least in the same tonal family, you'll look positively brilliant.

Great Shapes

Shapes come alive when mirrored in matching accessories. For example, you can mirror a circle-print scarf by wearing hoop earrings and a pair of shoes that have a circle clip, or a pair of sandals with straps joined by a huge circle on the vamp.

Patterns Benefit from a Coordinating Accessory

If you're wearing a herringbone cap, pair it with a herringbone clutch or muted herringbone stockings. Or, if you're wearing a pair of smashing fabric pumps in a flower print, clip a flower in your hair and another on your green suede tote.

Texture Loves a Friend

If you're wearing beaded pumps, add a beaded string evening bag or clutch to emphasize the richness of their texture. If your skirt is heavily embroidered, lightly textured spirals on a pair of shoes or stockings will knock their socks off.

Mixing Moods Has to Be Carefully Done

For a classic look, it's usually best to keep your accessories understated. Even if your painted artist overalls are sensational, pairing them with elegant sandals would rattle a few onlookers. Of course, that said, if you're mixing moods quite intentionally and have carefully thought out your choices, go for it!

Hosiery Is Tricky

When it comes to hosiery and shoes, it is far better to wear opaque stockings with sporty shoes, and nude looks (match the color to your inner arm) with dressy shoes. Limit patterns and avoid glaring contrasts, including cream or white. Tonal matches or ultra-sheer hosiery closest to your natural skin tone is the most flattering and most tasteful choice.

If you rebel against high heels take care to do so in a very smart hat.

George Bernard Shaw, playwright

special needs

Before we wrap this party up, let's address special needs. If you have special needs, as I do, you can still create a fabulous s*hoe attitude* and don the golden slippers. A close friend of mine, whose feet and ankles require the extra support of tightly laced boots, dealt with her limitation by creating her own style. She had a wardrobe of boots—light-colored ones for spring and summer, suede ones for fall, textured leather for winter, embellished ones for dressy affairs—all on flat rubber soles or 1-inch heels. Because wearing boots in the spring and summer, particularly in California, required panache, she assembled a wardrobe of clothes that made it work. She usually wore flowing, pale-colored, linen skirts with uneven hems (wool in winter), soft linen blouses (silk blouses or sweaters in winter), and long scarves or shawls. She looked simply magnificent, sexy, and fashionable. She created her own style. This is exactly what we are referring to when we discuss *shoe attitude*, girls, and you can do it too!

If you have special needs, buy the most comfortable, stylish shoes you can afford and punch them up through creative clothing and accessories. My feet, for example, do better in lace-up oxfords or tight boots, so I buy snappy ones. I have flat, navy blue fake alligator oxfords that look very smart with all my dressy trousers; a soft leather, black ankle boot (extra-wide) on a ½-inch heel (with an added rubber sole to soften sidewalk impact) for dressy slacks; and sensible fisherman's sandals in exotic leathers and bold colors for everyday wear. I found a pair of men's sneakers (extra-wide) in hot colors that are far more stylish than any wide sneakers I've seen in the women's department.

My niece, Michele, has been constantly challenged by the simple fact that her feet are longer than most. "Since I've worn a size 11 shoe since the age of 15, shoe shopping has been a lifelong nightmare. Even if a store carries a size 11, chances are the choice of styles is limited to two or three, and chances are the few pair they had in stock will already be gone. I often spend an entire day shoe shopping only to come home empty-handed. Until they joined me on shopping expeditions, friends with "normal" sized feet never believed me when I said I couldn't find a single pair of shoes to buy; when my boyfriend accompanied me, he was astounded by the challenge, and refreshingly sympathetic. It never takes me several hours to find a pair of great shoes; it takes me months to find a semi-decent pair of shoes.

"Online shopping has widened my prospects significantly. Often I will see a style I like and then search for the manufacturer to special-order the shoes. It ends up costing me a lot more than being able to buy shoes from a retailer, but it keeps me in cute shoes! I've also grown adept at spotting the lime green and orange dots shoe retailers will paste onto larger sizes during sales events, which minimizes wasted time while I shop.

"Finding shoes for work is especially challenging. When I found a pair of smart-looking black flats (½-inch heel and a small, gold chain across the vamp) for work, I wore them relentlessly, everywhere, with everything for two fall/winter seasons. They were actually a cute pair of shoes that fit my feet! Unfortunately, they gave up the ghost about four years ago, and I still haven't found the perfect replacement. However, I've now discovered an excellent cobbler, so when I do find the perfect pair, I'll be able to keep them forever!"

Having long feet or troublesome feet is not an excuse to forgo fashion and surrender your *shoe attitude*. Work a little harder, be creative, and forge your own distinct personality. Not only will you be much happier; you'll soon have others not only admiring your style, but copying it.

creative things to do with shoes

How your favorite shoes become art

Okay, girls, the hard work is all behind you; it's time to go a little wild. How about indulging your shoe obsession by literally turning your beloved shoes into art? For those of us who simply adore our shoes, here are some ideas for special projects that celebrate your obsession and bring the welcome breeze of whimsy into your home:

* Literally put special shoes on a festooned pedestal for proper adulation.
* Put pumps, mules, or sandals adorned with rhinestones, glitter, fur, etc., on a mirror and use them as centerpieces.
* Create a wall of fame by displaying your most outrageous shoes on mini-shelves mounted to a wall.
* Use witty, lightweight, miniature shoes to create a shoe mobile
* Photograph your favorite shoes, make heat transfers from the images, and use them to create T-shirts, place mats, pillows, etc. Extra credit for adding clever phrases!
* Convert your photos to sepia in your photo editing software, print them on beige-toned, lightweight paper, and decoupage

shoe obsession: open to all shoe-a-holics!

So, by now, you've established that you have an addiction. Don't worry, honey, you're not alone! Invite your shoe-happiest girlfriends over to celebrate your dependency over cocktails. Run your party like a 12-step meeting, with this exception: Right after each girl introduces herself, identifies her particular shoe obsession, and admits her sins, have two martinis and then quickly move into play. Ideas include:

- Sharing tales from the shoe rack.
  How about that salesman who literally drooled when he fondled your perfectly pedicured foot? Or the crazed woman who grabbed the last pair of Manolos right out of your hands? Or the teenaged fashionista who followed you around for two hours noting everything you picked up?

- Do know your designer?
  Match biographies, famous shoes, and styling habits with names.

- Name your poison.
  Create shoes diseases to explain your obsession. Describe symptoms, prognosis, and cure. A few examples:

  Park-insanes—You always wear stiletto heels, requiring your escorts to park three inches from any destination. Prognosis: incurable. Cure: buy smaller car.

  St-st-stiletto syndrome—You stand in front of shoe store windows for hours, stuttering. Exceptional cases involve clawing at the windowpane. Prognosis: incurable. Cure: buy the damn shoes!

  Shoe affective disorder—You suffer from chronic crankiness when deprived of desired footwear. Prognosis: not so good. Solution: buy luscious green suede pumps.

them onto furniture, hatboxes, flowerpots, and any other items you can think of. Extra credit for using textured paper!

* Photograph your favorite shoes or a sequence of favorite shoes, from baby shoes on up, and use photo software to create a poster showing your transformations through time. Print older photographs in sepia, and use ragged edges to jazz it up.

* Have your favorite shoes bronzed and use them as bookends.

* Create a shadow box to show off your wedding shoes, wedding invitation, sepia-toned photographs, veil, dried roses, garter, etc.

* Create a shadow box to house a loved one's baby shoes, rattle, booties, sepia-toned photograph, and other baby memorabilia.

* Create a shadow box using your favorite shoes, favorite hat, veil, gloves, stockings, ticket stubs, photographs, and other souvenirs to commemorate a special event, such as an anniversary, a night at the opera, first date, or prom.

* Fill a pair of stiletto-heeled pumps with bewitching massage oils, perfumes, feathers, or other sensual items and offer them as a present to your lover.

* Fill pumps, boots, or oxfords with dirt and use them as flowerpots; fill fun shoes with colorful sand or glass marbles and use them as memo holders.

Are you having fun yet?

okay, girls . . . start walking

Oh dear, you're so eager to shop, you're almost out the door! Before you go dashing off into your future, let's quickly review the six principles of *strutting your stuff.*

1. *Feet first*

Footwear choices do shape your life. Just like our shoe heroine, Cinderella, we've all learned that shoes do make the woman. Hopefully, you're determined to stand on solid ground and are already shopping for the *souliers* (dream shoes) that are going to catapult you into your brilliant future. Remember, shoes equal transformation!

2. *your shoe history*

Those saddle oxfords and ballet slippers you wore as a little girl may still hinder you and your shoe attitude. By examining your past, you have chased away any negative clouds that limited full expression of your blossoming personality. You have cleared the path for your new vision to manifest. Change is good, darling; now hurry along, and promise me that you'll forever banish dawdling!

3. *i think shoes, therefore i am*

Making decisions about your life and incorporating shoes into your action plan. Aren't you amazed at how taking a close look at the image you presented to the world has changed the way you feel about yourself? Simply keep shoes in the forefront of your image creation, and you'll be forever stepping out in style.

4. *out with the old shoes, in with the new you*

Change your shoes and jump-start your career and your love life. How lovely it feels to have literally chucked the worn-out shoes of your past and launched your re-creation! If you've done your homework, you're well on your way to expressing your true personality in all realms of your life, *and* exploring a few experimental detours just for fun.

5. *shoes make the woman*

   Revamping your shoe attitude to enhance your style, image, and life. Now that you've fostered the proper *shoe attitude*, you're breaking new ground in all areas of your life and loving it. You're using fashion statements to say to yourself and to the world that you are a woman who values her appearance, appreciates quality, changes with the times, and possesses the all-important *je ne sais quoi*.

6. *strut your stuff*

   Mastering Shoe Attitude. After laying all the groundwork, you created and instituted a concrete plan to revamp your wardrobe and more fully match your outer appearance with your inner beauty. Congratulations are in order! Now all you have to do is stay on the path, and you'll be beyond fine— you'll be positively, radiantly, confidently, and magnetically you.

Alas, our shoe odyssey has come to a rapturous end. I'm fully confident you have developed *shoe attitude* to the max, revamped your clothing, shoe, and accessory wardrobe, and learned how to *strut your stuff* in all aspects of your life. You've come a long way from the early days of unconsciousness and have metaphorically— and very importantly—removed the wooden shoes of your past and have skillfully, mindfully, and gleefully slid your feet into their golden slippers. It's time to reclaim your rightful heritage, live your design, and achieve your dreams. Don't be afraid; you're ready for the ball. Go now, and always remember: Every shoe that makes you feel like a princess is a golden slipper.

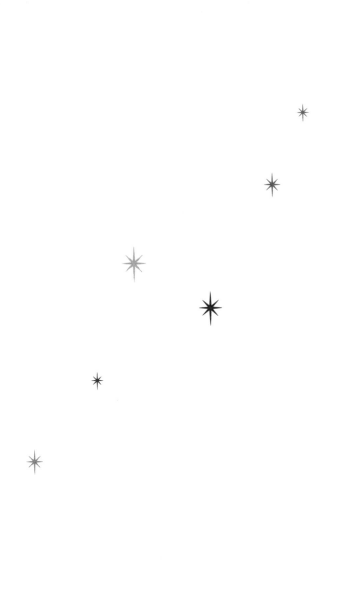

appendix

shoes and feet 101

before you go tripping off to the stores to build your new shoe wardrobe, I implore you to review the following basic information about feet and shoes. After all, protecting and nurturing your feet is what makes fashion exploration possible.

the nature of feet

As one might imagine—considering that they serve as the base of our operations and the engines of our mobility—feet are complicated, intricate bodily structures. Each foot contains 26 bones, 33 joints, 107 ligaments, 19 muscles, and several yards of tendons, all of which tightly knit your foot together and allow it to function properly. The 52 bones in your feet make up about one-quarter of all the bones in your body! The structure of the foot consists of the following:

* **Forefoot**: Five metatarsal bones and phalanges (toes) connected by multiple joints, supported by tendons and ligaments.

✳ **Midfoot**: Five to seven tarsal bones, the navicular, the cuboid, and three cunei. The midfoot meets the forefoot at the metatarsal joints.

✳ **Hindfoot**: The talus and the calcaneus form the heel. The talus rests on tops of and forms the pivotal, lower half of the ankle.

shoe components

The following parts create a shoe:

✳ **Last**. The foot replica that shoemakers use to shape the uppers. Lasts establish placement of the arch, which affects the distribution of weight and placement of your foot in the shoe. In the old days, wooden replicas were handmade and shoe uppers were hand-fitted to the last to ensure proper fit for each size. Hands-on designers, like Manolo Blahnik, are famous for hand-carved, individualized lasts specific to each design. Although automated, shoe factories still create lasts to use as guidelines, but lasts can vary greatly among factories and even among styles within the same factory.

✳ **Shank**. The curve under the arch that determines how the shoe supports the foot and how your weight is distributed. A correctly fitting shank will absorb your weight across both the ball of your foot and your instep. Strong metal shanks support your ability to walk long distances and reduce foot fatigue.

✳ **Quarter**. Where the back of the shoe meets the foot, wrapping around your heel. If the quarter is too high, it will cut into your ankle; if it's too low, it doesn't offer needed support.

* **Vamp**. The top of the shoe. Primarily aesthetic; however, a high-cut vamp, or a tightly laced vamp, offers valuable support by holding the foot in place. You absolutely do not want the vamp to cut into your flesh. A low-cut vamp can be highly seductive, creating what industry insiders call toe cleavage.

* **Toe box**. The area surrounding and holding the toes. The toe box's primary job is to adequately contain your toes, without cramping them. You can wear pointed-toe shoes as long as they extend well beyond your toes. If a toe box fits properly, it will allow all your toes to lie flat in its widest part. A wide and slightly elevated toe box will give your feet room to operate according to *their* design.

* **Heel**. Heel heights, widths, and materials can drastically alter your comfort level. Obviously, wider heels offer increased balance; lower heels offer increased comfort and proper positioning; rubber heels offer cushioning. Thanks to designers like Salvatore Ferragamo, who created a steel shaft to stabilize stiletto heels, we all can enjoy high heels in moderation. Simply alternate stilettos with low heels, or limit their wear to those occasions when limited walking is involved.

making sure the shoe fits

Obviously, as we learned from our poster girl, Cinderella, proper fit is crucial. Let's review some important tips for making sure the shoes you want to adorn your feet also fit your feet.

* Never automatically select shoes by the size marked inside the shoe. Shoemakers use a variety of shoe lasts, and sizes can vary greatly among shoe brands and styles.

* Select a shoe that conforms as nearly as possible to the shape of your foot. Don't kid yourself on this.

* Have your feet measured regularly. You may have been wearing the wrong size for eons; the size of your feet increases with age. Wearing properly fitting shoes permits your toes to stretch to their natural flattened state, and keeps a smile on your face.

* Have both feet measured. Most people have one foot that's larger than the other. It's important to fit the largest foot and add insoles or other adjustments for the smaller foot.

* Schedule your shoe fitting for the end of the day, when your feet are largest (and tired). If you're going to wear them with socks, bring along a pair; ditto with nylons.

* Stand during the fitting process and check to be sure that there is adequate length (an additional ⅜ to ½ inch, or the width of your thumb) for *your longest toe* (remember: your second toe may be your longest toe). Avoid lifting your toes, which gives an inaccurate measurement; instead, rock forward slightly and push down on the toe box with your thumb.

* Make sure the ball of your foot fits comfortably into the widest part (ball pocket) of the shoe. Your foot and the shoe should meet, greet, and bend in the same place.

* Don't purchase shoes that feel tight; stretching may ease the fit slightly but rarely works even minor miracles.

* Check the heel for comfort. Your heel should fit comfortably in the shoe with a minimum amount of slippage; the top edge of the shoe's heel (or quarter) should not hurt your ankle.

* Put on both shoes and walk around the store to make sure the shoes fit and feel right. Avoid thinking they will wear in. Well-fitting shoes are comfortable at the outset!

size does matter

The most important thing you can do when choosing shoes is to make sure that the widest part of your foot matches up with the widest part of the shoe. Flex your feet and make sure the shoe is bending in the same place as the ball of your foot. This measurement is far more important than the length per se. Surrender all vanity when it comes to size. If your feet will be more comfortable in longer shoes, buy longer shoes.

Wider toe boxes also promote foot health and comfort. If you wear shoes with toe boxes shaped to match your feet, your tootsies will thrive! While this may be a challenge when buying hot, hip shoes, the most comfortable, healthy shoe you can buy is one with a toe box that matches the shape of your foot as closely as possible. Of course we don't want to totally surrender pointed toes, but you can increase your foot health by buying them in a wide width or, if wide widths aren't available, buy them at least one-half size longer than your normal size.

wearing the right shoes at the right time

For all sporting or walking events, protect your feet by wearing broken-in athletic shoes or broken-in, super comfortable, substantial flats, preferably with arch supports and padding inside the shoes, as well as on the soles. For other occasions when you need maximum support and comfort, keep in mind the following:

* Oxford lace-ups support your feet far more than slip-ons.
* Leather shoes allow your feet to breathe and increase your comfort.
* Wearing a thin pair of cotton socks under a thicker pair of cotton socks will limit sliding, which tires feet and causes blisters.
* Thong, mules, and slip-on sandals offer limited protection, and also tire your feet and your calf muscles.

other commonsense basics

* Exercise your feet by walking. It not only works all those muscles and tendons in your feet; it also boosts overall health.
* Alternate shoes, particularly heel heights, regularly.
* If you adore high-heeled pumps and you're on your feet a lot, try walking pumps (shoes with an athletic construction, wider toe room, and reinforced heels). The American Orthopaedic Foot and Ankle Society evaluated a number of popular women's dress shoe lines in terms of beneficial heel design, toe room, slip resistance, comfort, cushioning, and breathability. Easy Spirit Jet, Aerosoles, Mocc A Rena, Dexter, Rio, Nine West Espy, and Hush Puppies Earl received high marks.
* If your feet hurt constantly, you may have a physical problem that needs to be addressed. Rather than self-medicating with over-the-counter pads, gels, or arch supports, ask your physi-

cian for a referral to a specialist, either a podiatrist or an ortho-
pedist, as appropriate.

✳ If you are diabetic, it is vital that you see a podiatric physician
at least once a year for a checkup! People who have diabetes,
poor circulation, or heart problems should not treat their own
feet, because they are more prone to infection.

For more information about foot structure and foot health, check
out the following Web sites or write directly to these agencies.

American Podiatric Medical Association (APMA)
Toll-Free: (800) 275-2762
www.apma.org

American Academy of Podiatric Sports Medicine
Toll-free (800) 438-3355
www.aapsm.org

American College of Foot & Ankle Orthopedics & Medicine
Toll-free (800) 265-8263
www.acfaom.org

American College of Foot and Ankle Surgeons
Toll-free: (800) 421-2237
www.acfas.org

bibliography

Andre, Mary Lou. *Ready to Wear: An Expert's Guide to Choosing and Using Your Wardrobe.* New York: Perigee Books, 2004.

Apeles, Teena. *Women Warriors: Adventures from History's Greatest Female Fighters.* Emeryville, CA: Seal Press, 2003.

Baudot, François. *Fashion: The Twentieth Century.* New York: Universe Publications, 1999.

Bettelheim, Bruno. *The Uses of Enchantment: The Meaning and Importance of Fairy Tales.* New York: Vintage Books, Random House, 1975.

Brenner, Marie. *Great Dames: What I Learned from Older Women.* New York: Three Rivers Press, 2000.

Chace, Reeve. *The Complete Book of Oscar Fashion: Variety's 75 Years of Glamour on the Red Carpet.* New York: Eye Quarto, Inc., 2003.

Dariaux, Genevieve Antoine. *A Guide to Elegance: For Every Woman Who Wants to Be Well and Properly Dressed on All Occasions.* New York: HarperCollins, 2003.

Duranko, Michael, and Penina Goodman. *Bootism: A Shoe Religion.* Kansas City, MO: Andrews McMeel Publishing, 2003.

Eldershaw, Jane. *Heart and Sole: The Shoes of My Life.* New York: St. Martin's Press, 2004.

Farr, Kendall. *The Pocket Stylist: Behind-The-Scenes Expertise from a Fashion Pro on Creating Your Own Unique Look.* New York: Gotham Books, 2004.

Feldon, Leah. *Does This Make Me Look Fat?: The Definitive Rules for Dressing Thin for Every Height, Size and Shape.* New York: Villard Books, 2003.

France, Kim, and Andrea Linett. *The Lucky Shopping Manual: Building and Improving Your Wardrobe Piece by Piece.* New York: Gotham Books, 2003.

Gilman, Susan Jane. *Kiss My Tiara: How to Rule the World as a Smart-Mouth Goddess.* New York: Warner Books, 2001.

Hall, Marian, with Marjorie Carne and Sylvia Sheppard. *California Fashion: From the Old West to New Hollywood.* New York: Harry N. Abrams, Inc., 2002.

Heard, Neal. *Sneakers: Over 3,000 Classics from Rare Vintage to the Latest Designs.* London: Carlton Books, 2003.

Johnson, Anna. *Three Black Skirts: All You Need to Survive.* New York: Workman Publishing, 2000.

Kinsel, Brenda. *Brenda's Bible: Escape Fashion Hell and Experience Heaven Every Time You Get Dressed.* San Francisco: Wildcat Canyon Press, 2004.

Kinsel, Brenda. *Brenda's Wardrobe Companion: A Guide to Getting Dressed from the Inside Out.* San Francisco: Wildcat Canyon Press, 2003.

Kinsel, Brenda Reiten. *40 Over 40: 40 Things Every Woman Over 40 Needs to Know About Getting Dressed.* Berkeley, CA: Wildcat Canyon Press, 1999.

Manheim, Ralph (translator). *Grimms' Tales for Young and Old: The Complete Stories.* New York: Anchor Press, 1983.

Mazza, Samuele. *Cinderella's Revenge*. San Francisco: Chronicle Books, 1994.

McDonough, Yona Zeldis (ed.). *The Barbie Chronicles: A Living Doll Turns Forty*. New York: Touchstone, 1999.

McWilliams, Tracy. *Dress to Express: Seven Secrets to Overcoming Closet Trauma and Revealing Your Inner Beauty*. Novato, CA: New World Library, 2004.

Meltzer, Carole Swann, and David Andrusia. *Feng Shui Chic: Change Your Life with Spirit and Style*. New York: Fireside, 2003.

Mogul, Stuart. *Perfect Feet: Caring and Pampering*. New York: Stewart, Tabori and Chang, 2003.

Munier, Paula. *On Being Blonde: Wit and Wisdom from the World's Most Infamous Blondes*. Gloucester, MA: Fair Winds Press, 2004.

Newman, Cathy. *Fashion.* Washington, DC: National Geographic, 2001.

Nicholson, JoAnna. *Dressing Smart for Women: 101 Mistakes You Can't Afford to Make and How to Avoid Them*. Manassas, VA: Impact Publications, 2003.

O'Keeffe, Linda. *Shoes: A Celebration of Pumps, Sandals, Slippers, and More*. New York: Workman, 1996.

Opie, Iona Archivald, and Peter Opie. *The Classic Fairy Tales*. New York: Oxford University Press, 1980.

Palmer, Gladys Perint. *Fashion People*. New York: Assouline, 2003.

Smith, Nancy MacDonell. *The Classic Ten: The True Story of the Little Black Dress and Nine Other Fashion Favorites*. New York: Penguin Books, 2003.

St. James Fashion Encyclopedia: A Survey of Style from 1945 to the Present. Detroit, MI: Visible Ink, 1997.

Stephens, Autumn. *Wild Women Talk Back: Audacious Advice for the Bedroom, Boardroom, and Beyond.* Boston: Conari Press, 2004.

Stover, Laren. *The Bombshell Manual of Style.* New York: Hyperion, 2001.

Taggart, Judie, and Jackie Walker. *I Don't Have a Thing to Wear: The Psychology of Your Closet.* New York: Pocket Books, 2003.

Tatham, Caroline, and Julian Seaman. *Fashion Design: Principles, Practice, and Techniques: The Ultimate Guide for the Aspiring Fashion Artist.* London, England: Barron's, 2003.

von Franz, Marie-Louise. *Interpretation of Fairy Tales.* Dallas, TX: Spring Publications, 1970.

Vreeland, Diana, et al. *D.V.* New York: Da Capo Press 2003.

Willdorf, Nina. *City Chic: An Urban Girl's Guide to Livin' Large on Less.* Naperville, IL: Sourcebooks, Inc., 2003.

Woodall, Trinny, and Susannah Constantine. *What Not to Wear.* New York: Riverhead Books, 2002.

about the author

Susan Reynolds has spent fourteen years in the shoe industry, more than seven covering fashion, features, and hard news for industry authorities such as *Footwear News*, sister publication to *Women's Wear Daily*, and *W* magazine, among others. Ms. Reynolds currently works as a freelance writer and photographer, and divides her time between Paris, New York, and San Francisco.

Readers are encouraged to visit *www.changeyourshoes.com*, where they can access Ms. Reynolds' Change Your Shoes Hotline and receive fashion tips directly from the source.